Unanswered Questions in Psychiatry

"This is a timely and important book. Psychiatry and mental health care are not progressing as expected. Joel Paris analyses ten fundamental problems and proposes pathways for their solution. Necessary reading for anyone concerned with patient care."

John Livesley, Professor Emeritus,
Department of Psychiatry, University of British Columbia

Unanswered Questions in Psychiatry

Joel Paris
McGill University

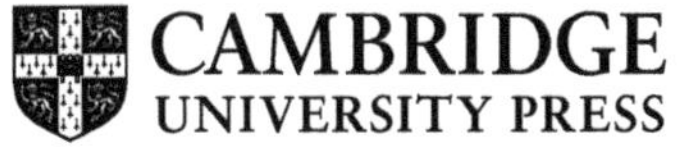

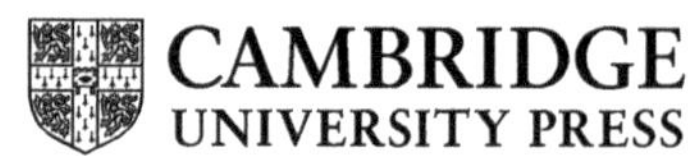

Shaftesbury Road, Cambridge CB2 8EA, United Kingdom

One Liberty Plaza, 20th Floor, New York, NY 10006, USA

477 Williamstown Road, Port Melbourne, VIC 3207, Australia

314–321, 3rd Floor, Plot 3, Splendor Forum, Jasola District Centre, New Delhi – 110025, India

Cambridge University Press is part of Cambridge University Press & Assessment, a department of the University of Cambridge.

We share the University's mission to contribute to society through the pursuit of education, learning and research at the highest international levels of excellence.

www.cambridge.org
Information on this title: www.cambridge.org/9781009653541

DOI: 10.1017/9781009653589

© Joel Paris 2026

This publication is in copyright. Subject to statutory exception and to the provisions of relevant collective licensing agreements, no reproduction of any part may take place without the written permission of Cambridge University Press & Assessment.

When citing this work, please include a reference to the DOI 10.1017/9781009653589

First published 2026

A catalogue record for this publication is available from the British Library

A Cataloging-in-Publication data record for this book is available from the Library of Congress

ISBN 978-1-009-65354-1 Paperback

Cambridge University Press & Assessment has no responsibility for the persistence or accuracy of URLs for external or third-party internet websites referred to in this publication and does not guarantee that any content on such websites is, or will remain, accurate or appropriate.

For EU product safety concerns, contact us at Calle de José Abascal, 56, 1°, 28003 Madrid, Spain, or email eugpsr@cambridge.org

....

Every effort has been made in preparing this book to provide accurate and up-to-date information which is in accord with accepted standards and practice at the time of publication. Although case histories are drawn from actual cases, every effort has been made to disguise the identities of the individuals involved. Nevertheless, the authors, editors and publishers can make no warranties that the information contained herein is totally free from error, not least because clinical standards are constantly changing through research and regulation. The authors, editors and publishers therefore disclaim all liability for direct or consequential damages resulting from the use of material contained in this book. Readers are strongly advised to pay careful attention to information provided by the manufacturer of any drugs or equipment that they plan to use.

To my students who pursued academic careers in psychiatry, and most particularly to David Goldbloom.

Contents

Acknowledgments

David Goldbloom, who was my student 40 years ago and went on to have a brilliant career in psychiatry, read an early version of this book and made many important suggestions for improvement.

Introduction

I.1 How I Became a Psychiatrist

Psychiatry has always had more questions than answers; it still does. But the mystery of the mind and its maladies is what attracted me to choose this profession. Like most clinicians, my aim was to help people suffering from mental disorders. I hesitated and made several false starts before committing myself to this career, but once I completed my training, I never looked back, and have only recently retired (after 52 years).

I have long been (and still am) a skeptic. I am suspicious of simple answers to difficult questions. As the American journalist HL Mencken (Wikiquote) once put it, "Explanations exist; they have existed for all time; there is always a well-known solution to every human problem – neat, plausible, and wrong." Thus, when less is known, ideas that are simple and dogmatic fill the gaps.

For me, the challenge of studying human behavior was irresistible. I was always interested in understanding the mind. Then, as a student at the University of Michigan, I took an introductory course in psychology, taught by a graduate student in a seminar. One day another student dropped by and asked if any of us wanted to spend a weekend as an observer at a nearby mental hospital. We ended up visiting there for about half a dozen weekends, observing patients and meeting with staff.

This was 1957, when antipsychotic drugs were just being introduced (in small doses). Thus, one could still observe patients paralyzed by catatonia standing like statues in the hallways, while paranoid patients spent days writing endless notes in dark corners. One young woman had spent over a year in hospital after making multiple suicide attempts. Fascinated with this world, I applied to medical school. I was accepted to McGill, which had a famous psychiatry department, and spent most of my life in Canada. (In view of the recent developments in the USA, my decision may have been prescient.)

In the 1960s, when I began my residency training, psychoanalysis dominated North American psychiatry. For some, even today, its theories offer a sense of certainty about mental illness, even if most of them are wrong. Its model attempts to explain almost anything about psychopathology, but it is not testable. Psychoanalysis is not an evidence-based discipline, but a collection of compelling anecdotes that claim to support a speculative set of hypotheses.

Why then did the psychoanalytic model flourish? The main reason was a lack of credible alternatives. Its main competitor at the time was behavioral therapy (BT), which I considered a nonstarter. The clinicians who developed the BT model were just as confident of the efficacy of their methods as psychoanalysts had been. But they made the fatal error of only measuring behavior, seeing the brain as a "black box" that could be ignored. This is why BT was eventually replaced by cognitive behavioral therapy (CBT), in which cognition became the main focus.

In the late 1960s, many of my teachers were psychoanalysts. I have spent the rest of my career showing why they were wrong. Even then, I viewed their model with skepticism and was seen as a rebel. But when I talked to colleagues trained in other traditions, I was perceived as "one of them." My early years in academia were dominated by a psychodynamic perspective. Then, nearing age 50, I gave up these beliefs. I undertook a conversion to the scientific model of evidence-based psychiatry. I am still a "born again" proponent of these principles. I have never again allowed myself to believe in theories based on clinical experience alone, or to lose my respect for empirical data as the best pathway to truth.

My own journey paralleled what was happening in my chosen discipline. Psychiatry has long been divided into biological and psychosocial models. Advocates of biological psychiatry see changes in the brain as central to psychopathology. They talk to patients, but do not offer talking therapies. Instead, they make diagnoses and prescribe medications. But decades after the "pharmacological revolution" of the mid twentieth century, treatment of mental illness with drugs remains in its infancy.

Our arsenal of interventions benefited most dramatically from new medications for severely ill psychotic patients, whose delusions and hallucinations rapidly disappear with treatment. But these drugs do not cure psychotic illnesses. Moreover, no one knew (or still knows) quite how and why they work. Finally, a narrow biological model lacks a coherent theory to explain why some fall victim to mental illness while others do not. (To be fair, this is probably true in medicine as a whole.)

The other side of psychiatry overlapped with clinical psychology, in which psychotherapy was the main treatment. My teachers espoused a model that they confidently claimed could be applied to a wide range of disorders that fail to respond to medication. I practiced and taught psychotherapy over the first decade of my career. Then, like so many before me, I became disillusioned. Some of my results were good, some were not so good, and most were middling. This inconsistency led me to a crisis that was only resolved when I returned to my background in medical science.

I became an advocate of evidence-based psychiatry and began a second career in research. I had a late start, but made up for it by publishing over 200 scientific papers and 30 books. I was now committed to facts rather than rhetoric. I felt comfortable asking my colleagues and students to back up their ideas with empirical evidence.

Another issue that troubled me early in my career was how psychiatry, when its practice was devoted to psychotherapy, was any different from clinical psychology. I wanted to make use of my medical training and knew how to prescribe medications. I suspected that many of my teachers were treating normal people with normal life problems, not patients with mental illnesses. I wanted to apply my skills to severely ill patients.

A friend of mine who had an academic career in medicine once advised me: "[E]very top doctor needs to be an expert on one disease." With this in mind, I developed a subspecialty in psychiatry that fit my wish to treat people who most required my services. I had always been interested in suicidal patients who present in emergency settings and hospitals. At the very least, these patients would be either alive or dead after therapy. But clinical psychologists avoided them, mainly due to fear of losing them to suicide.

The result was that I focused my career on the treatment of borderline personality disorder (BPD). This diagnosis has a history going back almost a century (Stern, 1938), but has always been controversial. Some of my teachers considered BPD to be fuzzy and unreliable, and advised me not to use this diagnosis. But I came to realize that I had been treating this disorder without recognizing it. Moreover, there is a role (albeit a smaller one) for medication in this population. This background allowed me to be comfortable in prescribing (and deprescribing) drugs. Given my training in medicine (a world where patients can and do die), I was in a better position than other professionals to manage chronically suicidal patients.

I continued to practice general psychiatry, where my skills could be applied to a wider range of patients. But I also needed to join a research community whose work could shed light on the etiology, outcome, and treatment of BPD. I only established myself as a researcher in my early fifties. I had to update my knowledge of statistics and research methods, but benefited from clinical experience as a consultant, a therapist, and a teacher. Half of my books are about personality disorders, while the other half focus on broader problems in psychiatry. All were intended to be read by practicing mental health clinicians. I have always felt validated when students and colleagues told me that my ideas resonated with their own experience.

1.2 What This Book Is About

The present book is a follow-up to an earlier one: *Fads and Fallacies in Psychiatry*, 2nd edition (Paris, 2022a). That book focused on some of the serious errors, past and present, that have plagued psychiatry since its beginning. I have also published a book titled *Prescriptions for the Mind*, which examines the current state of clinical practice (Paris, 2024). This book will, however, focus on the future. It will describe the most important unanswered questions about psychiatry and suggest what kind of research would be needed to address them.

Much of psychiatry remains mysterious, so I am not claiming that I can predict its future. To quote Isaac Newton (https://todayinsci.com/N/Newton_Isaac/NewtonIsaac-PlayingOnTheSeashore.htm), "I do not know what I may appear to the world, but to myself I seem to have been only like a boy playing on the seashore, and diverting myself in now and then finding a smoother pebble or a prettier shell than ordinary, whilst the great ocean of truth lay all undiscovered before."

I have heard it said that elderly psychiatrists write books about the future of their field; I am now one of them. There are many books about the practice of internal medicine and surgery, but one hardly ever sees books defending the validity of these domains. Psychiatry is the only specialty in medicine that has had to do so. It has even had to defend itself about the reality of mental illness. But psychiatry is too complicated for easy answers. That is probably why quite a few academic psychiatrists have written about the state of their specialty. Some are too congratulatory (Lieberman, 2015). Others have argued that over-valuing the manuals we use for diagnosis has distorted our research agenda (Frances, 2013).

I remember that when I was a child in the middle of the last century, pundits tried to predict the future of the next 50 years. Almost all turned out to be wrong. Building on advances in transportation earlier in the century, some predicted flying cars. Hardly anyone ever imagined the role of computers.

I have written this book from what I hope is a humble perspective. I will not propose, as others have, that technology will solve the problem of understanding and managing mental disorders, that reading the genome will support "personalized treatment," or that more powerful drugs are about to emerge to treat the most severely ill patients. I also doubt that we need any more forms of psychotherapy labeled by three-letter acronyms. We already have hundreds of them, and most are fundamentally the same. Finally, while my discipline has shown it can help troubled people, the belief that psychiatry should play a role in changing society is sadly mistaken.

Instead, this book will be organized around a series of *unanswered questions* that have important clinical implications for those who work with mentally ill patients. Psychiatry needs to be seen as a young and exciting field. I will focus on what kind of research is needed to address its problems. I will mainly recommend carrying out studies that measure biological and psychosocial risk factors in the same population. We also need much more longitudinal research that studies patients across the life course.

Meeting these goals will be expensive and require a good deal of patience. But these questions will eventually have to be answered, even if it takes another century to do so. As it stands, the most basic mechanisms driving mental disorders are still unknown. We need to know much more, but that will take time. There have been too many false promises that basic sciences are on the cusp of a breakthrough. This book will show why such predictions are unlikely. We have to accept that, given the fact that, with 86 billion neurons and trillions of synapses, the human brain is the most complex structure in the entire universe.

Here are the 10 major questions this book will explore:

(1) What causes mental illness, and what is the role of evolutionary forces, genes, neurobiology, life experiences, and social stressors?
(2) How should mental disorders be classified? Do we need a categorical system, a dimensional system, or both?
(3) Can adherence to a biopsychosocial model of mental disorders inform clinical practice?
(4) Do psychiatrists need to stop centering their practice on symptoms, and allow a more central role for personality traits?
(5) Is it possible to ensure a broad commitment among clinicians to evidence-based practice?
(6) Why is treatment with psychopharmacology, after dramatic advances 50 years ago, in a state of suspended animation?
(7) What is the role of psychotherapy in psychiatric practice, and should medical practitioners still be offering it?
(8) Why, in spite of extensive research, are psychiatrists unable to predict or prevent suicide?
(9) Do psychiatrists have a mandate to recommend how modern society could be made less stressful?
(10) What can we do to increase access to mental health treatment?

Each chapter will be devoted to one of these questions. Chapter 1 will examine the multiple interacting forces involved in mental disorders. None are sufficient by themselves, and in most cases, all are necessary. While biological risks lead to a *risk* for mental illness, they do not necessarily *cause* disorders on their own but have effects that are due to interactions with environmental risks. Similarly, adverse life experiences do not necessarily lead to mental disorders unless they interact with heritable risks. That is why most people are resilient to adversity, and why negative life events are most likely to affect a vulnerable minority.

This chapter will then review the current relationship of neuroscience to psychiatry. We have a better understanding of how genetics relates to psychopathology, but this domain of research is still at a very early stage. The same can be said for research based on neuroimaging. We have invested enormous resources in this domain, based on a hope to define mental illnesses as brain diseases. Some advocates do not even speak of psychiatry, but of "neuropsychiatry," and foresee a fusion of neurology and psychiatry into one specialty that focuses on disorders of the brain (Insel and Quirion, 2005; Taylor, 2013). These views are premature and deeply misleading.

While I have seen much progress in my lifetime, I am much more impressed with what is unknown than what is known. We have effective drugs for some illnesses, but do not know exactly how they work and what brain functions they target. That remains a project for the future. We need to be guided by a better theory. I will show that the hope that cognitions, emotions, and behaviors can be accounted for at the level of neurons is implausible. We need to study brain and mind at a more complex level.

A noted biologist (Theodosius Dobzhansky, Wikiquote) once said, "[N]othing in the life sciences makes sense outside the context of evolutionary theory." This chapter will review the role of evolution in psychopathology. But that point of view raises another question. If the main goal of any organism is to pass on its genes, why are human beings so often afflicted by mental disorders that make doing so more difficult? The answer requires us to understand that nature is not necessarily benign or progressive. There are major individual differences between individuals, some of which are of clear benefit, while others are beneficial in one set of circumstances but not in others, and still others are often harmful.

The alternate view, that life experiences are a main cause of psychopathology, while it has been downplayed by biological researchers, has had great influence on psychiatry and clinical psychology. This model has been largely debunked for severe mental illnesses, but it lives on in the construct of post-traumatic stress disorder (PTSD). As we will see, most people who suffer traumatic experiences do not develop PTSD, or mental disorders of any kind (Paris, 2023c). Resilience is the rule. Adverse life experiences can trigger mental illness but are not its main cause. *This having been said, severe stressors can also be risk factors for severe forms of mental illness.* Above all, we need to avoid separating biological and psychological pathways to psychopathology, and to treat casual pathways as one interacting system.

Chapter 2 will focus on how psychiatry classifies mental illness. Several systems are currently in use. As a practitioner in North America, I make use of the Diagnostic and Statistical Manual (DSM), now in its 5th edition (DSM-5-TR, American Psychiatric Association, 2022). In Europe (and in most of the world), the standard system is the International Classification of Diseases, now in its 11th edition (ICD-11; World Health Organization, 2018). I will also examine alternatives to these systems, which are based on quantitative dimensions instead of categories of illness.

Psychiatry has long struggled with how best to classify psychopathology. Given our limited knowledge about the causes of mental illness, how could it be otherwise? Medicine has usually seen illness as a set of categories. That model works well with a wide range of diseases that have biological markers and that can be treated in specific ways. Yet some medical illnesses (e.g., hypertension) lie on a dimensional spectrum, and can only be diagnosed when they pass a cut-off point.

Psychiatry and clinical psychology have used categories and dimensions for different purposes at different times. These research domains have a strong tradition of using quantitative data derived from self-report. Dimensions are particularly relevant when doing personality assessments. They are also favored by biological psychiatrists who find a lack of biomarkers in psychiatry, due to their being related more closely to traits than to categories of illness. But hardly anyone would suggest eliminating categories such as schizophrenia or bipolar-I, diagnoses that closely resemble medical illnesses.

This chapter will explore some of the debates about the DSM system of diagnosis used by many psychiatrists, particularly in North America. My view is that this system is better than its predecessors, but that, in spite of the best intentions, it mistakes symptoms for illnesses. I will also explore how the public, with the help of the internet, has used the DSM system for self-diagnosis, with troubling results.

Examples of these problems include seeing depression as one illness, diagnosing ADHD for inattention of any kind, and viewing life adversities as the one and only cause of PTSD. I will also show that the ICD-11 does not avoid the problems with the DSM system but repeats them. Finally, I will review the dimensional systems that have been proposed to replace categories in diagnosis and will show why they have serious problems of their own.

Chapter 3 will examine the biopsychosocial (BPS) model of psychopathology. It will show why this approach is more compatible with a scientific psychiatry than biology, psychology, or sociology by themselves. It will argue that problems in causation need to be addressed by an interactive model. This biopsychosocial approach has had its critics but is still the best way to move forward. Testing the model will ultimately require longitudinal research in large samples to measure biological, psychological, and social risk factors. This chapter will also identify problems with the idea of linear causation, which is reductionistic and ignores crucial ideas of complexity and emergence.

Chapter 4 will address the question of whether psychiatry focuses too much on symptoms and fails to understand the role of personality in psychopathology. If diagnoses in psychiatry can be slippery and somewhat misleading, what should clinicians target in treatment? Is it sufficient to focus on the symptoms for which patients seek help? Or should we also be concerned with the traits that underlie these clinical features?

Keep in mind that heritable traits have different effects in different environments. Thus, biological and psychological variability can lead to better chances of passing on one's genes, but that need not always happen. In psychology, we describe these differences as *temperament* or *personality*. These are heritable differences. Many are normal variations, but some are equivalent to losing in a genetic lottery.

Personality traits set a limit on the effects of standard treatments for symptoms. We have reasonably good tools for managing problems such as depression and anxiety, through medication and/or psychotherapy. Even so, only a little more than half of these patients obtain a stable remission. There is a good body of evidence indicating that personality profiles (especially high neuroticism, as well as diagnosable personality disorders) interfere with recovery. People who lack success in work and intimate relationships over long periods of time will have more difficulty with changing their personality. Many patients with "comorbid" PDs have only a fair response to either pharmacological or psychological treatment. Yet we now know that some personality disorders (especially BPD) are treatable with specialized forms of psychotherapy.

While psychiatry has sometimes been called a stepchild of medicine, personality and personality disorders might be called the stepchildren of psychiatry – acknowledged but not well loved. Personality profiles affect work and intimacy and are linked to more chronic psychological symptoms over the lifespan. Psychiatry has given these traits insufficient attention and needs to acknowledge that personality profiles can also require treatment.

Chapter 5 will examine the state of evidence-based treatment methods in psychiatry. It will show why the rise of evidence-based medicine has been a boon to the specialty. It is no longer acceptable for practitioners to rely on expert opinions based on ideology rather than data. However, we cannot assume that all practitioners are committed to evidence-based practice, as opposed to following their own ideas. Moreover, given that clinicians do not always have the time to update themselves on research, we need better ways to offer continuing medical education, without depending on pharmaceutical companies to inform (or misinform) us.

Chapter 6 will focus on the future of psychopharmacology. Are psychiatrists relying too much on medication and not making use of alternatives? The story of psychopharmacology is one of dramatic success over a period from the 1950s to the 1980s. Those of us who are familiar with the history of this research know that some of its greatest triumphs came from luck (e.g., antipsychotics from use in anesthesia, antidepressants from drugs for tuberculosis). Sadly, this research domain has been in stasis for some time. Many patients do not fully respond to drugs, and we continue to struggle with "treatment resistant" illnesses. The result is all too often futile attempts at polypharmacy associated with an unnecessarily large burden of side effects.

Chapter 7 will review research on the practice of psychotherapy. Why are talking therapies, long known to be as effective as psychopharmacology for many mental disorders, not used more often? This situation is puzzling, considering the large body of research supporting the efficacy of psychological methods in depression, anxiety, addictions, eating disorders, and personality disorders.

The main obstacle is cost. Human resources are more expensive than prescriptions. Also, psychotherapy tends to go on for too long. Research shows that most therapies work within a few months, and there is little evidence for additional benefits beyond six months – or at most a year. Like the psychopharmacologist who keeps adding more drugs, some psychotherapists offer endless therapy in the vain hope of a breakthrough.

For now, the identity of psychiatry depends on its links to neurobiology. We are considered experts in drug treatment, and fewer of us spend a great deal of time talking to patients. Psychotherapy may only come to mind in disorders where it has a definite advantage over medications. It would help if psychiatrists read more about research on this form of treatment, which is mainly published in psychology journals. It would also help if psychiatrists would more regularly collaborate on treatment teams with psychologists. Finally, it would help if medically trained clinicians were open to carrying a few complex patients in therapy to understand the challenges of this kind of work.

Chapter 8 will focus on the question of whether psychiatrists can predict who is at risk for suicide, or whether they can actually prevent fatal outcomes. When patients attempt or threaten to attempt suicide, psychiatrists are usually called in to consult. Yet while we can often make useful treatment recommendations, there is no evidence that these evaluations predict or prevent fatalities.

The reason is simple. Death by suicide is much more rare than suicidal ideas or attempts. That discrepancy makes for too many false positives. The vast majority of those with suicide attempts or suicidal ideation never kill themselves. Long-term follow-ups have developed algorithms for predictions of risk, but they fail to predict outcomes in any individual case. Thus, in spite of the many books and articles promoting suicide prevention in clinical practice, it is not evidence-based. The main exceptions are based on reducing access to the means of suicide. There will always be suicides, but when they happen, we need not hold ourselves to blame.

Chapter 9 will focus on the relationship between psychiatry and societal forces and social risks. It will question whether having clinical experience allows clinicians to prescribe for society. Psychiatrists are not trained to solve social problems, and there is no evidence to show that they can do so. Yet some, whether on the left or the right politically, have not resisted temptations to pontificate as public intellectuals.

This chapter will show, however, that social risk factors play a role in the risk for psychopathology (e.g., social defeat in immigrants, or social breakdown in indigenous communities). But our profession lacks hard data to show that psychiatric expertise can make a difference in preventing mental disorders at a population level.

Chapter 10 will examine the prospects for access to care for mental disorders. There is little point in advancing the field if mental health services are inaccessible to most patients. But difficulty of access remains characteristic of mental health systems.

A brief epilogue will end the book with a summary of what psychiatry needs to do over the next half century. It will take a cautious view, given that accurate prediction of the future is not possible. I am skeptical of the claim that neuroscience will be the main source of advances in treatment in the near future, but hope this will happen in the current century. In the meantime, I strongly recommend designing mental health systems that provide better access to a wider range of therapeutic choices. Doing so would allow us to treat patients more effectively, and would actually save money for mental health systems.

Chapter 1

What Causes Mental Illness?

*Unanswered Question #1: **What causes mental illness, and what is the role of evolutionary forces, genes, neurobiology, life experiences, and social stressors?***

1.1 A Historical Perspective

Since the birth of psychiatry as a medical specialty, clinicians and researchers have been searching for the causes of mental illness. A century later, we still don't know. We can identify risk factors for illness but cannot predict who will fall ill. Even so, we treat patients with reasonable success: Most psychiatric treatments are as effective as those in internal medicine (Leucht et al., 2012).

One of the puzzling aspects of psychopathology is how many patients who develop disabling symptoms have been well functioning in the past. Some mental disorders have prodromal symptoms that begin in childhood, and some patients have a family history of psychopathology. In those cases, we can describe statistical risks but cannot make firm predictions. Moreover, most severe mental illnesses become clinically apparent in adolescence or youth (Jones, 2013). But the onset of a mental disorder can come as a nasty surprise.

Several theories have been proposed to explain the time of onset of mental illness. The contenders include a hypothesis that adolescence is a time when synapses in the brain are heavily pruned (Germann et al., 2021), when there are notable changes in hormone levels (Graber, 2013), and when psychosocial stressors make relationships more difficult (Grant et al., 2014). But none of these risks explains why some are afflicted while others are not.

Consider, for example, this personal anecdote. In my first year at university, I lived in a dormitory. I was 16 years old, away from home for the first time, and in need of guidance. A senior student, then in his early twenties, was responsible for helping everyone living on the floor. I was shocked when he suddenly developed a severe mental illness – found in his room, naked and delusional, attempting to paint the walls. He then went on to receive a diagnosis of schizophrenia at a prominent psychiatric hospital. As far as I knew, this young man had never been previously ill. What could have caused this breakdown? Seventy years later, psychiatrists still have only a general idea as to what lies behind the disorders they treat.

A year later, I observed a mental hospital as it then was. Some might have been horrified by what they saw there. But I could not help being fascinated with this world of madness. I soon learned that clinicians who treat mentally ill patients were also struggling to find explanations for severe psychopathology. Some thought that abnormal neurotransmitters could be responsible. Another idea, often the view of psychoanalysts, was that mental illness was due to bad parenting. A few therapists were even emboldened to treat psychoses with psychotherapy, but they had no success, often making patients worse (Dolnick, 1998).

Psychiatry has always had a large gap between theory and practice. That is still the case. Some of its greatest breakthroughs in biological treatment have occurred by accident (Healy, 2004). The use of antipsychotic drugs began when a new antihistamine was found to calm psychotic patients. These new medications turned out to be one of the most dramatic discoveries in the history of medicine. Within a few years, when prescribed these drugs, most psychotic patients could be discharged after brief admissions. Large mental hospitals ended up being demolished (including the one near my undergraduate university, which once had 4,000 patients), or converted into research labs (as happened in Canada, where I studied psychiatry). It is true that medications tend to leave patients only partially remitted, and that inadequate funding of treatment in the community has often left them seriously adrift (Frances, 2013). But no one claims that long hospital admissions are still needed.

1.2 There Is More to Psychiatry than Psychosis

Most patients have disorders that are painful but not incapacitating. The most frequent condition in outpatient practice is what diagnostic manuals call a "major depressive episode." But major depression is not a single condition (Parker, 2005). It is a heterogenous mix of symptoms that varies from brief experiences of low mood to extended and disabling psychopathology (Spoelma et al., 2023). A minority of patients need to be hospitalized, but the vast majority have episodes that are much less severe (Cohen and DeRubeis, 2018). This variability raises questions about whether it is possible to find a single pathway to depression.

The Diagnostic and Statistical Manual of Mental Disorders, 5th edition, text revision or DSM-5-TR (American Psychiatric Association, 2022) advises us to make this diagnosis if depression lasts for at least two weeks. But that is a very short time span, uncomfortably close to normal reactions to losses. Variability in severity makes it unclear as to whether all "major" depressions are the same, and whether they are really major. Research has questioned whether all depressions are part of a single spectrum (Parker, 2005).

There are notable sex differences in the prevalence of depression, with a strong predominance in women. These differences are more broadly seen in internalizing disorders, including anxiety disorders and post-traumatic stress disorder (PTSD), while men have higher rates of externalizing behaviors such as substance use and crime. We do not know the reason, but women score higher in the personality trait of neuroticism (see Chapter 4).

What does treatment tell us about the nature of depression? Not as much as one might think. Antidepressants were discovered by accident (Healy, 2004), and the tricyclic group was originally thought to be another set of antipsychotics. It was only when specific serotonin reuptake inhibitors (SSRIs) came on the market that we had anything like "designer drugs."

Antidepressants are useful tools, especially when depression is severe (Parker, 2005). But they are being overprescribed to people who would do as well, if not better, with a course of psychotherapy (Cuijpers et al., 2020). Since talking therapy is not well insured, physicians (not only psychiatrists) offer antidepressants routinely to patients with almost any clinical features of low mood. But psychiatry has no cure for unhappiness (Horwitz and Wakefield, 2007).

Anxiety disorders, as a group, have a similarly high prevalence. Fear is even more prevalent than sadness (Horwitz and Wakefield, 2012). Anxious symptoms such as excessive worry or panic attacks can also accompany depressive episodes. This overlap is mainly due to the fact that our diagnoses are imprecise. Most have massive "comorbidity," that is, they overlap with other categories (Pincus et al., 2004). These fuzzy boundaries are an artifact of the DSM system, which lists similar criteria for different diagnoses. It does not mean that patients have two separate disorders.

We often treat patients with problems that are close to normality. One of our subspecialties is addiction psychiatry. Another is eating disorders. My own domain of personality disorders concerns a group of diagnoses that describe long-term problems in finding a direction in life and establishing meaningful relationships (Paris, 2015a). All these conditions are common, and respond best to psychotherapy, while medications are much less useful. But as long as talking therapies are difficult to access, the gap will be filled by prescriptions.

1.3 Does Neuroscience Account for Mental Disorders?

Physicians treat many illnesses with success and have greatly increased the human lifespan. Scientists send rockets and telescopes into orbit. So why can't we cure mental disorders? The answer is that the brain is much more complex than planets, stars, or space itself.

Yes, neuroscience is currently on a roll. We know much more about which brain functions are localized and which are not. But the regions devoted to thinking and consciousness are widely distributed and operate at a higher level of interaction (Fornito et al., 2017). Understanding neural connectivity is (and will continue to be) an uphill climb. I recently heard a brain scientist on a podcast state that he felt he was climbing Mount Everest but remained in its foothills.

Dynamic complexity systems are nonlinear and lead to emergent properties (Rust, 2025). This is a model that best fits brain disorders. Such processes cannot just be mapped as a "connectome." You could measure the activity of every synapse and still not have a clue what the brain is doing. The reason is that the environment usually determines what most neurons do. As long as researchers delude themselves with the assumption that psychiatry is nothing but an application of neuroscience (Insel and Quirion, 2005), we will never solve these mysteries.

Psychiatry, therefore, also is unwise to reinvent itself as a branch of neurology, as it originally was. I know how neurologists see patients (I have been one myself, very briefly). They are certainly experts in diseases in which (unlike psychiatry) one can measure change in specific brain regions. They order scans and tests to confirm diagnoses, even when they are unlikely to show anything new. But neurologists do not always have the skills in managing behavior, emotions, and cognitions that psychiatrists have. We are limited by the symptoms that patients report but are trained in skills that help us to talk to people in trouble.

Psychiatry is also different because it concerns the mind, not just the brain. I am not advocating dualism; that is a long-debunked idea. But the mind, although totally dependent on brain activity, is an *emergent* construct, whose properties exist at a different level. This makes psychiatry a unique discipline in medicine. Due to ethical considerations, psychiatry cannot be an experimental science. So it has had to depend almost entirely on systematic observations.

We do not know how the brain produces consciousness. But what is crucial to psychiatry that we have the capacity to make choices. Thus, in spite of claims to the contrary, minds have free will (Baumeister, 2008). This is because our species could not have survived without a cognitive capacity for agency when the environment presents conflicting choices (Mitchell, 2023). Those who claim that the laws of physics mean that determinism rules human behavior are applying the wrong model, one that sees the mind as a machine. Moreover, other animals have a degree of consciousness and free will (Baumeister, 2024). Even bacteria choose to approach food and to avoid danger.

Given the complexity of our brains, there have been no useful animal models of mental illness. Some of the attempts to create them have been dubious, such as mouse models of schizophrenia (Ang et al., 2021) or of autism (Silverman et al., 2022). Animals have emotions and thoughts, but live in the present, and do not have the mental disorders that humans do. The more complex the brain, the more it is at risk of malfunctioning.

Some psychiatrists hope that technological advances will overcome the limitations of current research. Two scenarios based on technology have recently gathered a fair amount of attention. The first is artificial intelligence (AI). Here the hope is that machine learning could sharpen diagnosis, guide treatment choices, and identify those most at risk for psychopathology (Monteith et al., 2022). The second is personalized psychiatry (Baune, 2019). The hope there is to address "treatment resistance," often seen in depression, by identifying biomarkers or changes in the genome, which could be linked to variations in neural connectivity. These goals remain elusive, at least for now. Psychiatry is too complex to be a servant of any technology, no matter how powerful.

1.4 Mental Disorders Are Complex and Do Not Have Simple Causes

Psychiatry has not benefited from attempts at searching for simple explanations of complex pathways leading to mental disorders. The problem is that our minds are structured to favor *linear* causation. We struggle to see the world as it truly is – an enormously complex set of *interactions*. That is why statistical analyses in research these days usually report multivariate analyses instead of univariate relationships.

The fact that multiple interacting forces shape the development of mental illness supports the need for a broader model. This book will argue that psychopathology is best understood as *biopsychosocial*. While biological vulnerability leads to a *risk* for mental illness, it does not necessarily cause disorders in the absence of environmental risks. Similarly, adverse life experiences do not necessarily lead to mental disorders, unless they interact with heritable risks that have a basis in biology. The environment is not just something that happens to us but reflects the choices we make. Moreover, negative life events do not lead everyone exposed to them to develop mental disorders, but mainly affect a vulnerable minority (Paris, 2022b). Fortunately, those of us born with good genes and who grew up in a supportive environment are more resilient to adversity. Thus, gene-environment interactions are the best way to understand psychopathology (Uher and Zwicker, 2017).

We can also benefit from considering the role of evolution (Del Giudice and Haltigan, 2023; Gilbert, 1995; Nesse, 2023). Individual differences in vulnerability are in part determined by genes. If these biological variations lead to better ways of managing environments, they will be passed on and become more frequent in a population (Dawkins, 1976). But if the main goal of any organism is to pass on its genes, why are human beings so often afflicted by mental disorders that make reproduction less likely?

The answer to this question is that nature is not necessarily benign or progressive. Natural selection is based as much on competition as cooperation. That is why many social scientists dismiss (or do their best to ignore) evolutionary psychology (Pinker, 2002, 2011). Many of them dislike competition and believe in social change on a road to Utopia.

Another key concept in psychiatry concerns individual differences in risk factors related to heritable traits. *Personality* is the construct that reflects these differences in vulnerability (Paris, 2022b). Trait profiles describe how individuals respond to and process life events, leading to major differences in personality. Some traits are of clear benefit. Others, such as neuroticism, are more problematic. Heritable traits also have different effects in different environments: They can be positive or negative in one set of circumstances but not in another. Temperamental variability remains in the gene pool because environments are not stable.

Genetics and environments interact in several ways. *Passive* gene-environment correlations occur when genes and environment mutually reinforce each other. *Active* gene-environment correlations occur when individuals seek out environments that align with genetic predispositions. *Evocative* gene-environment correlations occur when the environment reacts to genetically influenced behaviors. All these mechanisms amplify the effects of genes but are difficult to disentangle.

In summary, the biological factors in mental disorders carry a risk for psychopathology but are not its only cause. Keep in mind that brain sciences describe statistical risks, but do not fully account for outcomes. While a proverb says that "as the twig is bent, so grows the tree," the most lasting effects in development depend on gene-environment interactions.

1.5 Molecular Genetics

A few decades ago, at the height of excitement about the decoding of the genome, I chaired a committee for the recruitment of an endowed chair in schizophrenia. The donor was the father of a young man who had that illness, but died from complications of his medical treatment. The father, who kept up with media reports on science, had a hope for research to find a gene (or a small number of genes) that causes schizophrenia, and that this knowledge would lead to a cure.

The result of the search led to the hiring of a neurologist who was an expert in complex inheritance but had no expertise in schizophrenia. He continued his previous research for years without touching the problem of psychosis. The neurologist was later replaced by a PhD molecular biologist who also lacked clinical experience but was expert on neurotransmitters in mice. No doubt these recruits contributed to the advancement of neuroscience.

Many years later, I sat on a grant review committee and was told that there were now three or four mouse models of schizophrenia. I found the idea of an animal model for this complex disorder to be absurd. Mice do not suffer from psychoses, and we have no access to their thoughts. Not surprisingly, research using these reductionistic models has done little to help patients.

Schizophrenia remains as mysterious as it ever was. While errors in synaptic pruning are our best hypothesis for now, it is far from proven (Johnson and Hyman, 2022).

Can modern genetics untie this Gordian knot? The decoding of the human genome early in this century encouraged some people to expect that to happen, but this hope turned into another disappointment. Again, the obstacle to progress in understanding mental disorders lies in the complexity of the brain. Human beings have about 20,000 genes, fewer than many plants or animals. Most of their effects on heredity are not linear but arise from interactions with many other genes. The mistake was to believe that each gene has a specific function, or is "for" one outcome, such as physical or mental disorders. But that is only true for a small minority of Mendelian traits. (Even Mendel could not replicate his findings on peas when working on other plants.) It was eventually realized that almost all traits are shaped by large numbers of interacting genes.

For years, researchers searched for linkages on chromosomes and "candidate genes" that could be associated with specific forms of psychopathology (Farrell et al., 2015). That scientific program was a failure, and this line of research has now been largely abandoned (Turkheimer, 2024).

With this setback in mind, researchers adopted a different method called Genome-Wide Association Studies (GWAS). Here the idea was to read the entire genome in a large sample, searching for small variations at sites called single nucleotide polymorphisms. The results showed that innate differences are shaped by complex interactions between very large numbers of alleles. Thus, while almost all categories of mental illness have a notable degree of heritability, outcomes reflect interactions between hundreds of sites in the genome. Thus, genes work in teams, each carrying some aspects of the heritability of traits.

GWAS findings, by themselves, have not been strongly linked to any trait or mental disorder. A *polygenic risk score* can be calculated from GWAS data by adding up all associations with outcomes. But that procedure still only accounts for about 5% of the total variance (Plomin et al., 2022). Thus, the heritability gap does not disappear.

GWAS may turn out to be another failed research strategy. Turkheimer (2024) concludes that genes and environment are so closely intertwined that measuring them separately is impossible. How could it be otherwise in a science that aims to account for phenomena as complex as human behavior?

Research using GWAS also undermines the idea of offering patients "personalized medicine" based on their genome. You can pay companies to conduct analyses that claim to identify risks for various illnesses. But these relationships are purely statistical and not in any way reliable. Using such measures plays little role in uncovering the secrets of psychopathology.

The moral of this story, once again, is that innate differences are not direct outcomes of genes but are shaped by large numbers of interactions between them and with the environment. To understand mental disorders, we need to give up the hope for simple solutions and embrace complexity. Psychiatry is not near to doing so.

1.6 Behavioral Genetics

At this point, the best way to measure the heritability of psychopathology comes from *behavioral genetics*, that is, studies comparing the concordance of traits in identical and fraternal twins. These differences allow us to calculate heritability as a percentage in a population. The precise amount of variance that is genetic can still vary from one person to another. These findings have been consistently supported by another (but less common) method, adoption studies that compare traits in biological and adoptive parents (Kendler et al., 2018).

Turkheimer (2000) has proposed three "laws" of behavior genetics. The first is that all human behavioral traits are partially heritable, the second is that the influence of genes on human behavior is greater than the family environment, and the third is that a significant number of behavioral traits cannot be explained by either genes or the environment. When people are more similar because of being raised in the same family, one can speak of a "*shared environment.*" But the last two laws suggest that an "*unshared environment*" (outside families) is more important than growing up in a particular family.

So much for psychiatry's unfortunate history of blaming parents for every problem in their children! To put it another way, parents with one child believe in the primacy of the environment but change their minds once they have a second child. While the unshared environment can also include differences in experiences inside a family, siblings are generally quite different from each other (Harris, 1998).

Behavior genetics shows that all mental illnesses are under some degree of genetic influence (Giangrande et al., 2022). Some social scientists are skeptical about these conclusions, but they are biased against data that contradicts their own model. Uncertainty only lies in the level of variance under genetic influence. In the most T mental disorders (schizophrenia and bipolar-I), heritability can be as high as 80%. In common mental disorders (anxiety and nonpsychotic depression), the heritable influence is closer to 40% (Jang, 2005). Similar findings have been found in substance use disorder (Deak and Johnson, 2021), and a similar level applies to personality disorders (Jang, 2005).

Nonetheless, the heritability of these disorders has major clinical significance. Note that genes also have major effects on the personality traits that lie behind the symptoms of mental disorders (Turkheimer et al., 2014). These traits are risk factors for psychopathology, but do not necessarily predict the emergence of mental disorders (Smoller et al., 2019).

In summary, genes play a major role in all forms of psychopathology, but do not reliably determine its development. *This is also the case for schizophrenia.* Moreover, none of the illnesses we treat are related to just a few genes, but to very large numbers of them, each with a small effect. Finally, genetic risk factors cannot properly be understood without considering how they interact with the environment.

Genes are not only related to pathology; heritability is found in normal traits. These individual differences are described as *temperament* (in children) or as *personality* (in adults). Thus, personality emerges from an amalgam of genes and life experiences (Rutter, 2005). Some traits are beneficial, while others have little or no benefit. Even so, the same traits could have been functional in a different environment. Gene-environment interactions leading to feedback loops are what make traits problematic. This is why people at genetic risk may not consistently develop mental disorders.

1.7 Brain Imaging

Brain scans, particularly Functional Magnetic Resonance Imaging (fMRI), are a technology showing that different regions "light up" (i.e., are more metabolically active) when carrying out specific mental tasks. This kind of research is very expensive, and many publications using fMRI have been based on very small samples (Button et al., 2013), with results that fail to replicate (Turner et al., 2018). Moreover, given that connections are widespread across the brain, we may not really understand what we observe when a single region lights up on a scan.

When I trained in psychiatry, our ability to measure what goes on in the brain was limited to skull x-rays and electroencephalography. Imaging technology seemed at first to be a major breakthrough. Its methods began with computed axial tomography, later replaced by measures of blood flow and receptor binding to brain regions or positron emission tomography. The most common current method is fMRI. This method, focusing on specific brain regions, has been most widely used in research.

Researchers using imaging hoped to shed light on the *connectome*, that is, the way the brain is wired up (Fornito et al., 2017). One of the great questions in neuroscience has been the extent to which the brain functions as a whole, or whether specific regions carry out specific tasks. The answer is both. We know that some regions have particular functions, such as the role of the amygdala in fear, and of the hippocampus in memory. There are, of course, specific regions in the cortex that manage perception and movement. But vast regions in the frontal cortex are more related to "higher" functions such as cognition and consciousness. These networks are not necessarily specific but process how we learn from experience. Thus, even when we see a region of the brain lighting up on fMRI, these striking images are not a direct measure of the brain at work.

A psychiatrist specializing in addictions, along with a well-known psychologist, published a book titled *Brainwashed* (Satel and Lilienfeld, 2013) that focused on the hype around fMRI. Its main point was that the findings of brain imaging are at best approximate and do not provide a window to the mind.

Once again, we need not follow the advice of those who see psychiatry as nothing but an application of neuroscience, while downplaying the role of life experiences. A failure to consider interactions between heritable risk and life experiences is what has been called "psychiatry without the psyche" (Parnas, 2014). As for researchers who see psychiatry as a branch of neurology, their optimism is unjustified. These experts might be more cautious in their conclusions if they had more experience treating patients.

Brain imaging is a beginning. But we need better methods of measuring what goes on inside the "black box" under the skull. Perhaps future technologies will tell us more. In the meantime, we must be patient. Every few years, researchers tell us that we are on the cusp of a major breakthrough, but that has not yet happened. We remain on the cusp and may have to stay there for decades to come.

1.8 Neurotransmitters

Research in neuroscience has not solved the problems of psychiatry but it has revolutionized the biology of the brain. I can remember when this domain was in its infancy. When I was a student, models of how the brain works were illuminated by a theory of "cell assemblies" (Hebb, 1949), in which neuronal circuits followed the rule that "what fires together wires together." But the way these circuits (i.e., the connectome) function was not understood in any detail.

Serious attempts have been made by researchers to show that neurotransmitters malfunction at synapses in severe mental disorders. A Swedish scientist won a Nobel

Prize for his work in this domain (Carlsson, 2001). But these findings did little for the treatment of psychiatric patients. This line of inquiry has drawn criticism for being reductionistic and lacking a capacity to make predictions (Moncrieff et al., 2023).

The upshot is that while we still prescribe antipsychotics, antidepressants, and antimanic drugs, and have theories about their mechanism of action, we do not really know how they work in the brain. A lack of precise knowledge is not unusual in medicine (consider that we long lacked explanations for why aspirin reduces pain), but it is pervasive in psychiatry.

We need not be discouraged – just humble. Again, consider that the human brain is the most complex structure in the known universe. It is worth restating that it has circuits involving 86 billion neurons (and even more glial cells), all linked by trillions of synapses. While some parts of the brain are specific to certain functions, much of its circuitry is spread over different regions that work together.

A popular theory that has had a long sway over psychiatry, and is still supported by some experts, has been that many patients suffer from a "chemical imbalance." The most common neurotransmitters in the brain are glutamate, which is excitatory, and gamma-aminobutyric acid (GABA), which is inhibitory. But the most widely researched transmitters (serotonin, dopamine, acetylcholine, and norepinephrine) are neuromodulators that act as regulators across many regions. The largest body of research has focused on serotonin and dopamine, which are active in all parts of the brain.

However, consistent relationships between neurotransmitters and psychopathology remain unclear. Moncrieff et al. (2022), in an influential review, documented the lack of evidence for chemical imbalances in mental disorders, especially for serotonin. Initial findings told a story of high expectations that led to dead ends. While millions have been spent on this line of research, it has failed to find these chemical imbalances and has also failed to replicate findings that made this claim. This is why I always taught students not to rely on any single research paper. They need to wait until there is a meta-analysis combining results from multiple research groups. (Even then, the conclusions of meta-analyses can change when further studies appear.)

Do *interactions* between neurotransmitter activity and the environment do a better job at predicting psychopathology? For example, two much quoted papers over two decades ago found that a history of childhood adversity combined with low serotonin levels can be a risk factor for depression (Caspi et al., 2002), and that low levels of a mono-amine oxidase inhibitor can increase the risk for antisocial behavior (Caspi et al., 2003). These reports have been widely cited because, unlike most biological research, they seriously attempted to measure gene-environment interactions. However, these findings have been difficult to replicate, and the strength of these relationships remains controversial (Munafò et al., 2009). One major limitation of this line of research was that it examined single alleles, and not the genome as a whole.

In a famous paper titled "Why Most Research Findings are False," IoannIdis (2005) pointed out that *most* research in medicine fails to replicate. Often no one bothers to attempt replications. Medical journals may reject submissions that show when previous findings fail to do so. When replications have been carried out, some of the most cited research turns out to be false.

There are several reasons for this problem. One is that since scientific journals prefer to publish positive findings, negative results may never be submitted for publication but may end up in a file drawer. Another is that medical research is too often limited by sample sizes that are too small to prove anything. Still another is that samples in clinical research, even if they have adequate power, usually consist of volunteers for clinical trials who are not representative of clinical populations. Some of these problems can be dealt with by meta-analyses. But we need to realize that if even some of the most quoted findings in medicine and psychology are false, we can truly speak of a "replication crisis" (Ioannidis, 2012). That is why combining the results of many studies is so crucial.

1.9 Trauma and Adverse Life Experiences

I was taught by psychiatrists who took it for granted that the origins of mental disorders lie in an unhappy childhood. Even today, many clinicians (and their patients) continue to believe that early life experiences are the main cause of psychopathology. This idea, now folded into incorrect interpretations about the effects of trauma, retains a strong influence on psychiatry and clinical psychology. It does not consider that when the environment of childhood is problematic, it tends to stay that way, leading to cumulative effects from multiple exposures.

These ideas were even more extreme in the past. Early adversity was offered as an explanation for *severe* mental illnesses, even including schizophrenia (Pietrek et al., 2013). The assumption was that the earlier the trauma, the more severe must be the disorder. Actually, there is no evidence to support that idea, and quite a bit of evidence that contradicts it (Rutter et al., 2007). Moreover, the findings that have been quoted to support this hypothesis are only *correlations* that fail to distinguish between genetic and environmental risk factors.

In any case, explaining mental disorders as the result of single risk factors is almost always wrong. As research on the effects of life events on later functioning has consistently shown (Rutter, 2013), multiple hits have cumulative effects, while single events, even the most serious adversities, do not necessarily cause disorders.

1.10 Trauma and Psychopathology

Ideas about the purely psychological origins of psychopathology are less popular today. But they live on in the construct of PTSD. I am not questioning the validity of this diagnosis, even if its boundaries are not well defined (McNally, 2003). But I am concerned about the overdiagnosis of PTSD and the overuse of childhood trauma as an explanation for mental disorders. In the absence of longitudinal follow-up data, these attributions tend to be glib and mistaken.

The effects of trauma are by no means predictable. The vast majority of those who suffer traumatic experiences (at least 90%) will not develop PTSD or any other mental disorder (Paris, 2022c). This reflects the ubiquity of resilience in both community and clinical populations. The precise percentages of PTSD vary greatly depending on the nature of the trauma, with rape having the highest rate of 20% (Scott et al., 2018), while exposure to combat in war has a prevalence of about 15% (Stein et al., 2002; True et al., 1993).

By and large, exposure to trauma leads to PTSD in about 5–10% of cases. These relationships have also been documented in longitudinal research, following people who are most exposed to trauma, such as police, firefighters, or soldiers (McNally, 2003). Those who do develop PTSD are genetically vulnerable, either by personality traits associated with anxiety and depression such as high baseline traits of neuroticism (increased sensitivity to adverse life events). Notably, *all* the individual criteria in the DSM manual that define PTSD have a heritable component (Stein et al., 2002).

The studies that have examined people whose occupations put them at risk for exposure to traumatic events also has the advantage that follow-up begins prior to exposure and does not depend on memory. Most findings show that most exposed individuals never develop PTSD, but that those who do, have high levels of trait neuroticism and/or a history of mental disorder (McNally, 2003).

Similarly, several large-scale studies that followed children exposed to abuse into adulthood support a similar conclusion: Only a small percentage of long-term outcomes are related to childhood trauma (Fergusson et al., 2008; Paris, 2022c). Thus, the idea that trauma, by itself, can cause PTSD or related disorders is seriously misleading.

A better explanation lies in a trait called *differential sensitivity to the environment* that applies to most, if not all, life experiences (Belsky and Pluess, 2009). A similar concept is that of a "sensitive child" (Aron et al., 2012). It is worth noting that differential sensitivity also makes people benefit more from positive live experiences.

The personality trait that is most consistently related to PTSD is neuroticism. Moreover, those who develop PTSD may also have traits that make them more likely to be exposed to stressors, such as risk-taking (Stein et al., 2002).

The idea that early adversities are more pathogenic for children than for adults is based on the assumption that children are more emotionally dependent. But research has not found differences in levels of resilience to adversity between children and adults (Rutter, 2013).

In assessing trauma during childhood, consider that the way we remember the past is shaped by how we function in the present. Unfortunately, therapists who believe in the primacy of trauma are all too quick to encourage patients to report adverse early experiences and to explain their current difficulties on that basis. It would be hard to find anyone who has never had serious difficulty at some point during childhood. Some traumatic events, like sexual abuse by a caretaker, are much more pathogenic, but even children with the most severe life adversities do not necessarily develop mental disorders as adults (Fergusson et al., 2008; Rutter et al., 2007).

Failure to understand these relationships has led to serious overestimates of the prevalence of what is called "trauma," broadly defined to include adversities of all kinds (McNally, 2005). This is an example of *concept creep*, that is, how constructs in psychology tend to expand over time (Jones and McNally, 2022). For example, childhood emotional neglect is more common in clinical populations, and is not the same thing as abuse or trauma. I am not talking about families that do not offer even a minimum of care, but those in which the emotions of children are dismissed without providing support (Linehan, 1993).

An excessive focus on traumatic life events has led to false conclusions about its role in adult psychopathology. More longitudinal research is needed here. What it shows thus far is that resilience, not pathology, is the usual outcome of adversity. Most children, even when they grow up in a problematic environment, can still function well in adulthood. Those who do not have traits that make them more sensitive to their environment are relatively protected from developing psychopathology.

Thus, much of the research on trauma and life adversity is biased and misleading. As a clinician, I have seen thousands of patients with major histories of childhood adversity. But studies of community populations put these clinical observations into a different perspective. Trauma has a context, which includes everything from genes and brain systems to families and neighborhoods. Once again, we always need to consider the importance of gene-environment interactions. This is not to say that we should not work with patients with trauma histories, or fail to understand how adversity affects them, but that we should not attribute all aspects of mental dysfunction as related to adverse life experiences.

Unfortunately, an exclusive focus on trauma, associated with the prescription of "trauma-informed" therapy, has been adopted by some therapists and their patients. These methods, focusing on the processing of traumatic events, have not been shown to be superior to standard therapy for PTSD (Paris, 2022c). Trauma is a popular idea because it implies that psychological symptoms are someone else's fault, a point of view that can reduce stigma. But a focus on trauma leads to another set of conclusions that are mistaken. One best-selling book claims that trauma is somehow remembered in the human body (van der Kolk, 2015). Evidently many patients are searching for answers to problems, and trauma sells, in this case in an attractive package of pseudoscience.

In short, well-meaning therapists treating people with childhood adversity are making the same mistake as biologically based clinicians who see psychiatry as an application of neuroscience. They are searching for single causes of mental disorders instead of framing them within a biopsychosocial model. This bias leads to treatment choices that are less than optimal.

1.11 A Different Way of Looking at Environmental Effects

A large body of research has found that life adversities of all kinds, early in life or currently, are associated with mental disorders, both in adults and in children (Rutter, 2006). But these are statistical relationships in populations, not in individual patients. For this reason, we need to consider these findings in the context of a biopsychosocial model. Adverse life events cause mental disorders when there is also a prior biological vulnerability and/or stressful experiences that are multiple, long-standing, and cumulative.

To support this argument, I am drawing on the seminal work of Michael Rutter, a British child psychiatrist who conducted large-scale research programs and wrote influential reviews about gene-environment interactions in development (Rutter, 2006). He was also known for studies of the mechanisms, both biological and psychosocial, that drive resilience (Rutter, 2013). Moreover, he carried out with longitudinal research projects on children, including a landmark study of Romanian orphans who suffered severe neglect in infancy, but did well when adopted into British families (Rutter et al., 2007).

Rutter helped to define child psychiatry in the UK and was unique in an ability to straddle the gaps between genes and environment. Let me summarize his overall conclusions about the role of the environment in mental disorders (Rutter, 2005):

(1) Environmentally mediated risks have been demonstrated for the family rearing environment, peer groups, schools, and community.
(2) However, children have effects on parents, just as parents have effects on children.
(3) Associations with disorders can derive from the effects of a difficult child on family functioning.

(4) Individual differences in response to adversity are partly based on strengthening (or weakening) experiences prior to exposure, protective influences, and positive turning-point experiences.

(5) Behavioral genetic studies show that the unshared environment has more impact than the shared environment, but that does not mean that families have no impact.

(6) The main risk for antisocial behavior associated with "broken homes" is a function of family discord and conflict, rather than family breakup.

(7) The risks for depressive disorders in adult life are a function of impaired parenting, rather than of parental loss.

(8) Shared environmental effects are more prominent causes of antisocial behavior than for depression.

Rutter was a role model for me, although his eminence and originality far exceeded my own accomplishments. He followed children into adulthood to see what happened to them, and found that when the environment changed, so did children who had mental symptoms. He showed that resilience is ubiquitous, but that larger numbers of adversities have the capacity to overwhelm the "psychological immune system."

Rutter was not alone. Jerome Kagan was an American developmental psychologist who made a long scientific journey from psychodynamic theory to the biology of temperament (Kagan, 1998). His research showed how temperamental extremes, observable in infancy, shape traits in adolescence, and most likely in adulthood as well. Rutter and Kagan were part of a larger group of researchers pioneering a new paradigm called developmental psychopathology to build a bridge between biology, psychology, and the social context (Cicchetti, 2023).

In a systematic review of this research literature, Pine and Fox (2015) concluded that while the majority of mental disorders begin in childhood, they are not due to trauma alone but also due to interactions between heritable traits and environmental risks. They found that neurodevelopmental and psychotic disorders are most strongly associated with genetic variations due to temperamental variability, while gene-environment interactions create pathways that most strongly affect emotional disorders such as anxiety and depression.

These conclusions have not been changed by more recent findings. An interactive point of view makes it possible to think about genes and environment as a single system. You just need to stretch your mind.

1.12 Prospects for Understanding the Causes of Mental Disorders

The less that was known about the causes of mental disorders, the more theories there have been, with a tendency for explanations to multiply over time. Many advances in pharmacological treatment have occurred without understanding the etiology of the mental disorders for which they are used. But in view of the current lengthy hiatus in this domain of research (see Chapter 6), we probably need to know much more about causation.

The greatest triumphs of modern medicine have occurred in understanding acute illness, with the best examples being infectious diseases. The germ theory of disease was the breakthrough that eventually allowed treatments that can be managed by antibiotics or prevented by vaccination.

Chronic illnesses are a problem for physicians in all specialties. These conditions can be controlled, but tend to be resistant to cure. That is the situation for most of the problems that bring people to psychiatrists. But chronicity is usually a sign of complexity. No simple theory of causality is sufficient to understand the pathways to mental disorders.

To sort out these complex factors, we need longitudinal studies of children and adults in large samples, applying valid measures of biological risk and environmental risks. One way of doing this is to follow cohorts of monozygotic and dizygotic twins, and/or a birth cohort. Researchers in the UK (Fisher et al., 2015) and in New Zealand (Belsky et al., 2020) have been doing this for some time. But the problem of measuring the impact of genes and environment and their interactions is too complex to yield a clear verdict any time soon.

Answer to Unanswered Question #1
Mental disorders are complex and have multiple causes. Most are related to heritable vulnerabilities that are amplified by adverse life events. The biological aspects of this vulnerability are not currently explicable by specific changes in genetic makeup or in brain functioning. We lack a model that can accurately predict why people develop mental illness.

Classification

Unanswered Question #2: How should mental disorders be classified? Do we need a categorical system, a dimensional system, or both?

Ideally, medical diagnoses should be rooted in the causes of psychopathology. But as psychiatry is far from understanding the etiology of mental disorders, we cannot be sure of the validity of its diagnoses. Unlike much of medicine, we have no biomarkers to validate categories. Moreover, mental disorders have multiple causes at different levels, and their risk factors are not specific to particular symptoms or diagnoses. One of psychiatry's most leading researchers (Kendler, 2016, 2019) advises us to accept uncertainty and avoid oversimplifying complex pathways to causation.

Despite these obstacles, making diagnoses remains a clinical necessity. The reason is that psychiatrists need to communicate about psychopathology. Thus, their only real choice is to classify disorders on the basis of symptoms that patients report. But doing so does not make diagnoses valid.

The best-known current system, the Diagnostic and Statistical Manual of Mental Disorders, 5th edition, text revision (DSM-5-TR; American Psychiatric Association, 2022) does not have adequate reliability, even for depression (Regier et al., 2013). Much the same can be said about the International Classification of Diseases, 11th edition (ICD-11; World Health Organization, 2018). For these reasons, these systems can only be temporary, to be replaced at some later point by a classification based on etiology.

Unfortunately, diagnoses have a way of taking on a life of their own. The DSM manuals have always cautioned that they are not a guide to treatment. Clinicians *may* think otherwise. Hardly anyone pays attention to this caveat, or even knows it is there. Moreover, patients these days are self-diagnosing after consulting the internet, or what has been called "Dr. Google."

Clinicians often treat the DSM as what has been called the "bible of psychiatry." But this manual is not anything like a bible. When the DSM-III was published in 1980, it was so different from previous editions that the psychiatrists at my hospital feared being left behind, and we met in a weekly study group to bring ourselves up to date. The main innovation was the use of algorithms to guide diagnosis. Later editions made less radical changes. Even so, after DSM-5 was published (and met with heavy criticism), I was asked several times to speak about it and wrote a book offering my own take on that version (Paris, 2015b).

I concluded that the best one can say for the DSM manual is that - [WPQD3E 3N EQWH] as Winston Churchill once said about democracy – it is the worst system, except for any of the alternatives. It is neither a bible nor an encyclopedia. It is a distillation of current expert opinion, based on the work of committees.

We need to keep in mind that a diagnostic manual is only a tool. I have taught DSM diagnoses over the last four decades, largely because it offers a shorthand for communication. I tell my students to use the manual, but not to believe in it. But I am not sure they take my advice.

2.1 The Role of Diagnostic Manuals in Classification

The official manual of medical diagnoses (by treaty across the world) is the ICD-11. It is the official system for classifying mental disorders. But the ICD is less often used by psychiatrists in North America, where the DSM continues to be dominant. However, all codes for categories in one manual can be translated to those in the other.

Both the ICD-11 and the DSM-5-TR define each category of disorder based on clinical symptoms. The descriptors in ICD-11 allow clinicians to use their own judgment about whether patients meet enough criteria to make a diagnosis, while DSM-5-TR requires them to follow algorithms and count how many criteria are necessary. (Mostly this means more than half, but some categories can only be diagnosed if one specific feature is present.) Another difference is that functional impairments are considered mandatory in DSM-5-TR, but not in ICD-11. Even so, only a few disorders are present in one system and not in the other. Unlike DSM, the ICD system has not attracted as many controversies. However, one major change in ICD-11 is the replacement of categories of personality disorders (PDs) with dimensional measures. That issue will be discussed in Chapter 4.

Why does North America adhere to a different diagnostic system from the rest of the world? One reason is American exceptionalism. The USA is the only country that still measures temperature using the Fahrenheit system instead of the Celsius system that is standard in the rest of the world. Another reason is that a very large amount of research in psychiatry has, at least up to now, been carried out in the USA.

The DSM system needs to be understood in the context of its history. Born in crisis, when psychiatry seemed to be under siege, it endured in spite of criticism from all sides. While DSM is still the subject of active controversy, it is difficult to find researchers or clinicians who do not use it, even if they have reservations about its validity.

2.2 Distinguishing Mental Disorders from Normal Variations

One of the thorniest problems facing classifications of mental disorders is the fuzzy boundary between normality and pathology (Frances, 2013). In medicine, no one argues about diseases with well-defined biomarkers. But in psychiatry, the brain remains something of a "black box." There are no well-established biomarkers for mental disorders. But at what point should symptoms or behaviors be considered signs of pathology? It remains a judgment call. As underlined by Frances (2013), and by two recent books from the UK (O'Sullivan, 2025; Santhouse, 2025), we live in a time of overdiagnosis and diagnostic epidemics.

Paradoxically, a serious stigma is associated with psychopathology of all kinds (Corrigan et al., 2015). Many, if not most, people feel threatened by a label of any psychiatric diagnosis. I have also found stigmatic views to be common among physicians who are not psychiatrists – at least until they, or a member of their family, develop a mental disorder. When patients suffer, they and their families may have to overcome their fear of stigma and embrace a diagnosis that explains what they are going through.

Is there any agreed-upon way to define mental disorders that make sense for both clinicians and their patients? The most influential has been the construct of *harmful dysfunction* (Wakefield, 2007). In this model, deviance from norms leads to significant harm as well as decreased functioning, defined by an inability to carry out life tasks required by human evolution. Wakefield has had his critics, but no one has come up with a better alternative. The DSM system also requires the presence of clinically significant distress or impairment in social, occupational, or other important areas of functioning. But determining what is "clinically significant" remains a judgment call. *Similarly, the term "harmful" is not very precise, and effects can vary in different sociocultural contexts.*

We live in a time when experts and received wisdoms of all kinds are being questioned. Psychiatry has sometimes been seen as a defender of the status quo, with its patients as victims. Beginning in the 1960s, American psychiatry came under attack from two political directions. Right-wing libertarians such as Szasz (1960) saw psychiatry as a threat to individual freedom. Left-wing social scientists attacked psychiatry for making diagnoses that were nothing but social constructs (Foucault et al., 2013). Both sides criticized psychiatry for an inability to distinguish between normality and psycho-pathology. And both sides were hostile to psychopharmacology in any form.

In the past, a good deal of evidence showed that psychiatric diagnoses can be unreliable and idiosyncratic. For example, patients with psychoses were diagnosed as schizophrenic in New York, but as manic-depressive in London (Gurland et al., 1970). (After the introduction of lithium, the British preference for bipolar diagnoses was taken up by American psychiatrists.)

To add to these critiques, a famous study published in the journal *Science* (Rosenhan, 1973) claimed that researchers pretending to have mental illnesses were easily admitted to hospitals and given diagnoses of schizophrenia. According to the article, admission was triggered by reporting hallucinations, accompanied by paranoid ideas. Decades later, this study was found to be a fraud invented by Rosenhan himself (Cahalan, 2019). He seems to have been the only person who actually went into hospital, and none of the others have ever been found.

This supposed critique of psychiatric diagnosis must be one of the most successful frauds in the history of science (Scull, 2023). It has only now been exposed – but not before it was quoted in almost every textbook of abnormal psychology over the next 50 years. It says something about the lack of public confidence in psychiatry that it took half a century for the real story to be uncovered.

But since psychiatry was under attack, the American Psychiatric Association decided it needed a new diagnostic system to protect the profession. The two previous editions of DSM had offered descriptions of disorders that were vague and unreliable. This lack of validity led to a decision to develop a new manual (DSM-III, American Psychiatric Association, 1980) based on different principles. The process of writing a new DSM was directed by Robert Spitzer, an American psychiatrist with a strong sense of mission.

DSM-III required clinicians to use algorithms to make diagnoses based on sets of criteria that can be counted – with the hope that diagnoses made in this way would make them more reliable, making research into their validity possible. It was assumed that these categories would eventually be better defined by biomarkers and would then have a specific description that could be used to guide treatment choices. That is not what happened. None of these goals were ever met.

So what *did* happen? First of all, although most psychiatrists and clinical psychologists bought a copy of the DSM manual and kept it in their offices, they did not necessarily use it as intended (First et al., 2014). A busy practice promotes shortcuts, and few clinicians could remember all the diagnostic criteria in the DSM (typically 9 or 10 for each of several hundred categories). Most rarely opened the book to count them. Instead, clinicians focused on one or two criteria they saw as prototypical and made diagnoses much as they had before.

Decades later, it was found that even the most often used diagnosis in the manual, major depressive disorder, has a surprisingly low level of reliability (Regier et al., 2013). That should not have come as a surprise, since major depression is heterogeneous, lacks biomarkers, and does a poor job of predicting treatment response (Hollon, 2024; Parker, 2005). Even so, this diagnosis has long been used to support the routine prescription of antidepressant medications.

A flawed diagnostic manual is still better than chaos and guesswork. Thus, DSM-III filled a gap. It was a bestseller, as clinicians in the US and Canada, both inside and outside psychiatry, adopted the system. European countries continued using ICD in clinical settings, but academic publications often preferred the DSM. The one domain where the manual is carefully followed has been in research, where reliability is required for all measures.

But DSM or ICD manuals cannot address the most serious problems with classification. Their criteria for diagnosis are not based in science, but on clinical observations bolstered by expert consensus. The algorithms, written by committees, often reflected compromises between contrasting points of view.

In spite of the hopes of those who revised the manual, most categories were heterogeneous mixes of symptoms that are hard to separate from other diagnoses. This overlap between diagnoses has been called *"comorbidity."* This term is misleading. In fact, almost every category has broad comorbidity (McGrath et al., 2020). Most patients meet criteria for more than one diagnosis due to overlaps in their criteria – but not because they have two disorders. Comorbidity is an artifact of a provisional system, not a bible (Paris, 2015b).

One way to account for widespread comorbidity is that many illnesses fall on a *spectrum*. This point of view is appealing, particularly for psychologists who usually favor quantitative over qualitative data. But in practice, the spectrum concept has the potential to make a bad situation worse in that more people meet criteria, further amplifying overdiagnosis (Paris, 2020a).

Consider some examples. Autism is a neurodevelopment disorder that has long been known but considered rare. But since it was expanded in DSM-5 into a broader frame as autism spectrum disorder (ASD), this diagnosis has been made much more frequently both in children and adults (Fombonne, 2023; Mottron, 2021). It has reached the point that any child or adult with unusual levels of shyness and social awkwardness may be diagnosed with ASD.

Another example, which has sparked an even more formidable diagnostic epidemic, is attention-deficit hyperactivity disorder (ADHD). That increase was due in part to a change from hyperactivity in children to a wider spectrum seen at any age. I will return to this problem later in the chapter.

An even more worrisome example of defining spectra on the basis of symptoms alone, has been the practice of some clinicians to diagnose patients who have mood swings of any kind as falling within a bipolar spectrum (Paris, 2009b). My concern is that these diagnoses lead to unnecessary and potentially harmful use of medication. Most patients with mood swings do not have hypomanic episodes but have personality disorders that make them highly sensitive to their interpersonal environment. If diagnosed as falling in a bipolar spectrum, they will not be offered psychotherapy but prescribed antimanic drugs. This shows how misidentifying a symptom can lead to the wrong treatment.

One of the main proponents of a bipolar spectrum was Hagop Akiskal, formerly editor of the *Journal of Affective Disorders*. Twenty years ago, I was invited to debate him at a New York meeting of the American Psychiatric Association. The event was held at Radio City Music Hall, which was packed. It did not help that the moderator, Fred Goodwin, coauthor of a large book on bipolarity (Goodwin and Jamison, 2007), was clearly on Akiskal's side. Over time, this practice became less common. But other equally dubious categories have taken its place.

As the theoretical climate of psychiatry changed, the DSM system became part of a powerful trend to move closer to biological models. Psychiatrists aimed to be "real doctors" like other specialists, identifying disease categories and treating them with medication. But that remains only a hope for the future, not what the manuals tell us. We have come a long way from the view that diagnoses do not matter. They are not quite "real," but as long as they are a useful tool, that is good enough for now.

2.3 The Rationale for Dimensional Diagnosis

A more radical approach to the classification of psychopathology would be to replace categories with scores based on patient reports of symptoms and their severity. That is called *dimensional* diagnosis, because it yields data that supports quantitative spectra, as opposed to discrete categories.

Biologically oriented psychiatrists have long observed that biomarkers of any kind are more closely related to broader traits than to diagnostic categories (Mackay et al., 2009). This is another reason DSM algorithms are confounded by massive levels of "comorbidity" (Pincus et al., 2004). Again, the term only means that symptoms cross the diagnostic boundaries described in manuals.

Personality traits are a test case for the use of dimensions. These traits are an example, as they can be defined as characteristic patterns of thoughts, feelings, and behaviors that are relatively unique to individuals (Widiger, 2015). Psychologists trained in trait theory argue that categories tend to be artificial, and that information is lost when they are used to describe psychopathology (Krueger et al., 2018). Most think that a quantitative approach to diagnosis would be better.

So why has psychiatry not taken that advice? There are three possible reasons. First, radical revisions every decade or so undermine the perception that the current system retains a degree of validity. Second, there needs to be evidence that any major change in the diagnostic system actually benefits patients (Zimmerman, 2021). Third, and most important, if medicine continues to use categories, what would happen to psychiatry if it rejects diagnosis and goes its own way? Most likely, doing so would lead to a further estrangement from medical colleagues. The few dimensional measures in general medicine, such as hypertension, are the exception and not the rule. And would such a scenario be helpful for patients who are already stigmatized for being mentally ill?

2.4 Research Domain Criteria

Thomas Insel, former head of the National Institute of Mental Health (NIMH) in the USA, was a prominent critic of DSM-5. Arguing that "psychiatry deserves better," he promoted an alternative diagnostic method called the Research Domain Criteria (RDoC; Insel and Cuthbert, 2015). He proposed that the NIMH needed to meet the challenge of developing a diagnostic system that would be even *more* firmly rooted in neuroscience. This expectation came partly from the priorities of a US president who declared a "decade of the brain" to encourage research.

But there is still a striking lack of progress for developing a diagnostic system based on brain mechanisms. After decades of work, current research is just not up to the job. While basic neuroscience continues to progress, patients do not receive better outcomes due to its findings. We could manage almost as well with the treatments we had 50 years ago.

The RDoC system is a radical attempt to solve this problem. It is a matrix of scores claiming to be based on genes, molecules, cells, circuits, physiology, behavior, and self-reports. The system is much more theoretical than practical. But RDoC aimed to be a guide to research, not to treatment (Cuthbert and Insel, 2013). Its scores, organized as matrices ranging from brain science to social science, are too vague to be useful in practice. It is more of a manifesto for a reduction of human behavior to the activity of neurons (Paris and Kirmayer, 2016). Over more than a decade, there is no evidence that RDoC has had any effect on mental health care. The NIMH still mainly supports neuroscience, not projects to provide better care for the mentally ill, or to improve access to treatment. This is what happens when experts are convinced that mental disorders are brain disorders.

Insel (2022) eventually had second thoughts, acknowledging that well-funded biological research has failed to help most patients under our care. Psychotic patients can still end up being homeless, and rates of suicide and addiction in the US population remain higher than in other developed countries. Insel (2018) has tried to develop ways of monitoring patients to prevent suicide, as a kind of "personalized psychiatry." I will explain in Chapter 7 why that program is unlikely to succeed.

The main reason for the failure of RDoC to deliver better care lies in the immaturity of neuroscience. I have heard from my students that they were told by faculty in medical school not to train in psychiatry, on the grounds that research on the brain would soon solve all its problems. But we have now been waiting for decades – and are still waiting.

Some proposed solutions to these problems could make matters worse. I have already stated my opposition to making psychiatry into a clinical application of neuroscience, and returning to being a branch of neurology, as it was in the 19th century (Insel and Quirion, 2005). Yes, mental illness derives from the brain, but that is not why psychiatry is a separate specialty. Instead, it remains separate because it requires an entirely different set of clinical skills.

The view that mental disorders are brain disorders also implies a rejection of advances in evidence-based psychotherapy and undermines collaboration with the clinical psychologists who provide most of those treatments. Neuroscience is only *one* of the basic sciences for psychiatry. Unfortunately, medical students and residents are not being told that psychology and the social sciences are not as important for our specialty as biology.

The main problem with RDoC is that it fails to deal adequately with the psychosocial factors in mental disorders (Paris and Kirmayer, 2016). Putting these pieces together may take a long time, but a scientific strategy of reductionism to a neuronal level is bound to fail. It is not appropriate for psychiatry, which concerns complex phenomena with emergent properties. Moreover, the RDoC system has received only weak support from empirical data. It is just another bridge too far, of which we have already had too many. The proposal is a dead end and is little but another form of a "bio-bio-bio model" (De Rosa et al., 2018). The RDoC system has not gained traction since it was first proposed, and Insel, the psychiatrist who initiated it, has moved on to look for solutions through technology.

2.5 The HiToP Model

Another ambitious dimensional model proposed to replace current diagnoses of mental disorders is the Hierarchical Taxonomy of Psychopathology (HiToP). HiToP also offers a matrix of symptoms that can be scored but that are closer to clinical observation than RDoC.

At the top of the HiToP hierarchy is a general measure of psychopathology, called the psychopathology or *p*-factor (Caspi et al., 2014). At the next level of the matrix are diagnostic spectra (e.g., internalizing, externalizing, and somatoform symptoms). The next level describes "dimensional syndromes" that have a family resemblance or overlap. There are no diagnostic categories in this system.

I would like to be sympathetic to the ideas behind HiToP. But like most dimensional models, it offers a serious oversimplification of the nature of psychopathology. Yes, many disorders overlap and can be part of a spectrum. But that does not prove that similar symptoms have the same cause. Progress with classification will remain stalled until we discover the secrets of etiology.

The HiToP system currently remains of interest only to a highly motivated group of researchers and has not thus far attracted serious interest from clinicians. It has not been helpful in a search for the biomarkers that should underlie diagnostic spectra. I also worry that an emphasis on spectra could mean that we could further overestimate the prevalence of mental disorders. Paradoxically, this system would not necessarily lead to greater precision, but to overdiagnosis and diagnostic epidemics.

We can also consider here one other alternative to standard diagnosis: *network theory* (Borsboom, 2017). This point of view does not invoke either categories or spectra, but simply tracks the links between symptoms, "nodes" that track a shared vulnerability to several forms of psychopathology. Thus, network theory does not escape the problem of being grounded in symptoms instead of causal mechanisms. This model, like RDoC and HiToP, has thus far been mainly of interest to researchers (Stein et al., 2022).

2.6 Overdiagnosis and Diagnostic Epidemics

I see many problems with the current state of diagnosis in my specialty. But I do not support critics who hate *everything* about psychiatry. One example is the book *Mad in America* (Whitaker, 2001), now the basis of a website and a podcast. Founded by a journalist with limited scientific training, this movement finds little good to say about our profession. As far as I can tell, Whitaker rejects psychopharmacology and believes that psychiatrists are prescribing useless antipsychotic drugs that only do harm, especially in the long run. These views file in the face of an enormous body of evidence. I stand with the academics who want to make psychiatry better, not to destroy it.

To be fair, drawing a line between distress and disorder remains a real problem. And the problem of overdiagnosis is getting worse, not better. When the DSM-5 was published in 2013, many leaders in psychiatry were critical. Allen Frances, who had been the editor of the fourth edition, was disillusioned by psychiatric diagnoses applied to normal problems, and by the role of the pharmaceutical industry in promoting medications for life's vicissitudes. That is why he titled a book *Saving Normal* (Frances, 2013). He wants psychiatry to put aside its dream of a triumphal biological model for hundreds of disorders, and to concentrate on providing better services for severely and chronically ill patients. And unlike Insel, Frances supports a biopsychosocial model, favors evidence-based psychotherapy, and is critical of epidemiologists for having inflated the prevalence of mental disorders (Frances, 2014). Similar critiques apply to the diagnosis of major depression, as opposed to normal sadness (Horwitz and Wakefield, 2007), and to anxiety disorders, as opposed to normal fear (Horwitz and Wakefield, 2012).

Using the DSM system, half of the general population will meet criteria for at least one mental disorder over the course of a lifetime (Kessler et al., 1994). But do disorders with mild or temporary effects belong in a manual? Modern medicine does not exclude minor forms of pathology from its domain. But it does not follow that highly trained specialists should focus their efforts on patients with disorders that can be managed by other professionals. Once problems are coded in a manual, classifications tend to *reify* diagnoses in psychiatry.

Frances (2013) noted that the American Psychiatric Association (APA) made enormous profits on the various editions of the DSM manual, and that many of the experts on its committees were in the pay of industry. He concluded that professional organizations such as the APA have too many conflicts of interest to be trusted with the task of classifying mental illness.

The experts behind the ICD-11 have some of the same problems. The World Health Organization does not make money from publishing diagnostic manuals, which are available for free online. But I have been to conferences in Europe where luxurious wining and dining was paid for by the pharmaceutical industry, suggesting that the same dangers face psychiatry around the world. Fortunately, planning for the DSM-6, which will be published sometime in the next decade, is now excluding experts who have been compromised by overly close ties to the pharmaceutical industry.

Meanwhile, our lack of valid biomarkers for mental disorders opens the door to overdiagnosis, and a near-universal use of psychopharmacology. In this scenario, clinicians seize on a trendy category believed to be treatable and find it in a large percentage of their patients. The result can be dramatic changes in prevalence that can be called a *diagnostic epidemic* (Frances, 2013). Today we see many patients who self-diagnose (or who "diagnose" their family members) with whatever is the latest fad.

Some of these epidemics overdiagnose rare syndromes with doubtful validity. One example is multiple personality disorder, now called dissociative identity disorder (DID; Paris, 2019). This diagnosis is now widely regarded as an artifact of suggestion from therapists who convince patients they have repressed memories of traumatic events (McHugh, 2008; McNally, 2005). Supposedly, this process explains why some patients report having "alters," that is, other personalities. But these phenomena are almost always created by therapists asking leading questions. This diagnostic fad peaked in the 1990s and is less prominent today. Its current decline could be due to the fact that some of the therapists who promoted DID and treated patients for it were successfully sued and/or lost their license to practice.

DID is unique in that in spite of being built entirely on a fantasy, it has never been removed from the DSM. This is because the "experts" who sit on its committees are those who believe in its reality. As long as dissociative disorders are listed as a separate group in DSM, textbooks have felt forced to include a chapter on these dubious diagnoses, providing them with unjustified validation.

2.7 Overdiagnosis of Bipolar Disorders

Episodes of overdiagnosis tend to be based on expansion of existing and well-studied categories. Thus, diagnosis becomes more frequent in an attempt to simplify complex clinical phenomena, and to apply similar forms of treatment.

Let us return to the example of bipolar disorders (Paris, 2012). There are two forms: bipolar-I, which requires full manic episodes, and bipolar-II, in which only hypomanic episodes are present. (Documentation of hypomania, preferably confirmed by family or friends, is important because establishing how many days an episode has lasted can be tricky.) Bipolar-II (hypomania without mania) describes mood swings that need to be continuous for at least four days (but usually longer). Yet patients with other diagnoses also have mood swings. The fad for bipolar-II was based on the idea that a four-day cut-off was arbitrary (which is true). But advocates of a bipolar spectrum seemed to think that *all* mood swings, even those lasting for a day or a few hours, fall within the same domain.

It can be a mistake to diagnose bipolarity in patients who have unstable mood without mania (which is usually psychotic) or hypomanic episodes. Mood swings are by no means specific to bipolarity and often reflect emotional dysregulation. That helps explain why patients with borderline personality disorder (BPD) do not benefit from lithium or from antiepileptic drugs called "mood stabilizers," such as lamotrigine or valproate (Paris, 2020c, 2025). Notably, patients with personality disorders can have mood swings that last for hours, usually in response to interpersonal stressors.

Here an overdiagnosis of bipolar-II is based on a wish to successfully treat patients with unstable mood. The main motivation behind the bipolar fad was to prescribe anticonvulsive drugs, as well as lithium, that are useful for bipolar patients. As a consultant, I have seen quite a few patients who took these medications for years without benefit, but who continued because their physicians warned them that stopping would be dangerous.

One would think that patients would not want to have a severe mental disorder that can last a lifetime, as opposed to a personality disorder that usually remits over time. In fact, not all patients embrace this point of view. When people are afflicted with a serious illness, they may prefer a severe diagnosis that seems to explain their suffering – particularly if medication is believed to be a cure. Moreover, like their patients, clinicians can make a doubtful diagnosis because they want to prescribe a specific treatment. They are further encouraged to do so by the concept of a spectrum. The idea was that milder mood swings are a form of bipolarity that can be treated in the same way as classical mania or hypomania confuses symptoms with diagnoses. Most of these patients have a personality disorder with brief mood swings that can be managed by specialized psychological treatments.

The diagnosis of BPD has become more accepted in recent years. The reason is not only the large amount of research on this diagnosis. What has made the difference is the development of newer and more specific forms of treatment, particularly dialectical behavior therapy (DBT; Linehan, 1993), which have been shown to help most of these patients. Such cases have long been a major challenge to psychiatrists, which helps explain why they may be given other diagnoses, leading either to pharmacotherapy or to generic forms of psychotherapy.

2.8 Overdiagnosis of Attention Deficit Hyperactivity Disorder

A second example of overdiagnosis is attention deficit hyperactivity disorder (ADHD) in adults, a diagnosis that has now become epidemic (Gascon et al., 2022; Paris et al., 2015a). Some estimates of the prevalence of adult ADHD in the community claim that 10–15% of psychiatric outpatients have this disorder (Adamis et al., 2022), and that its community prevalence is 15% (Rowland et al., 2013). How is it possible that psychiatry missed all these cases for over a century?

We first need to ask whether ADHD is a mental disorder or an evolutionary mismatch (Swanepoel, 2024). In the latter case, it may be a set of traits evolved to support risk-taking behaviors, as opposed to sitting at a desk in an office. Many people have trouble focusing, especially at school or a job, that reflects changes in modern society. A lack of focus can also be the result of anxiety or depression (Castaneda et al., 2008).

It is hard to be sure of the validity of an ADHD diagnosis, particularly in adult patients, given that like other mental disorders, it lacks biomarkers. Neuropsychological testing is the best we can do, but its results are lacking in specificity (Holst and Thorell, 2013; Sawaya et al., 2024). In any case, testing is very expensive unless patients have generous insurance. Although ADHD patients have some differences on brain scans (see meta-analysis by Cortese et al., 2012), we do not know if they are specific or related to causality. It is also notable that ADHD patients have a wide range of comorbidities, particularly for substance use and personality disorders (Cumyn et al., 2009).

The less well defined a category, the easier it is to overdiagnose it. ADHD has undergone a major journey into "concept creep" (Haslam, 2016). I can remember when this condition was only based on hyperactivity, and when diagnoses were only made in children. But with time, ADHD was no longer limited to a hyperactive subtype, and a much broader spectrum of inattentiveness was added. And it was also found that ADHD can continue into adulthood (Adamis et al., 2022). It can be argued that inattentiveness is less disruptive than hyperactivity, and therefore less visible. But since lack of focus on tasks can be due to a range of other mental disorders, or be a variation of a normal trait, this change, along with changing the age of onset from 6 to 12 years, has led to overdiagnosis of the disorder (Batstra and Frances, 2012).

At least half of all children with ADHD retain some of these symptoms well into adulthood (Sibley et al., 2022). But that observation fails to consider that ADHD may be a mismatch with the demands of modern society (Swanepoel, 2024). In a large-scale birth cohort followed into middle age, people with ADHD symptoms in adulthood did *not* have a childhood history, raising the question as to whether later onset cases represent a different syndrome (Moffitt et al., 2015). Finally, as concluded by a Cochrane report (Boesen et al., 2022), the evidence for treating adult ADHD with stimulants is relatively weak, particularly in the long run, and its long-term effects have not been thoroughly researched.

But once a diagnosis is accepted into standard manuals, it becomes more prevalent in clinical practice. And as ADHD is being diagnosed more often, the prescription of stimulants has gone up accordingly (Olfson et al., 2013). Again, inattention and lack of focus are not specific to the diagnosis, and can be found in other conditions, including anxiety, depression, and personality disorders (Ribasés et al., 2023). And while ADHD diagnoses may seem to be confirmed to some extent by neuropsychological testing, results are often ambiguous.

The most common error leading to overdiagnosis is the absence of a childhood history of the disorder. In previous editions of the DSM manual, ADHD was described as a neurodevelopmental disorder that must begin before age 7. That requirement was extended to age 12 in DSM-5. A childhood onset is what one would expect from a disorder of this kind. In contrast, if symptoms only begin in adolescence, they will not meet diagnostic criteria. This means that a full clinical assessment requires an accurate history of behaviors in childhood. But our memories of the past are colored by our present mental state.

Our patients, many of whom spend a good deal of time online and/or have friends who encourage them to self-diagnose, may arrive convinced they have ADHD. The main reason for patient demands for this diagnosis is a belief that all you have to do to focus better is to take a stimulant. Once on these agents, unless side effects get in the way, patients can stay on medications for years. We do not know if those who continue to do so in middle age are at risk for cardiovascular effects of long-term use of drugs related to amphetamine (Docherty and Alsufyani, 2021). While patients can feel better on these agents, it is hard to rule out placebo effects in the short term, and a fear of stopping in the long term. Finally, it is not widely known, but long observed, that stimulants increase focus in normal people who do not have ADHD (Rapoport et al., 1978). In some ways, stimulant medications are becoming a normal part of modern life. Few of us use amphetamines, but a majority will take a morning dose of caffeine for a similar effect.

Research on ADHD needs to examine the fuzziness of the diagnosis, instead of downplaying or failing to assess the requirement for a childhood onset. Patients may insist that they had these symptoms but were not treated. Clinicians can ask to see report cards from primary school, and during childhood, and can ask parents and teachers to fill out rating scales. Adult patients may state that other members of their family have the same disorder. But that conclusion is rarely based on hard data.

ADHD has more validity as a mental disorder in children. But if diagnostic guidelines are not followed, the adult population will inevitably be heterogeneous. A recent finding that adults diagnosed with ADHD tend to die younger than average (O'Nions et al., 2025) made headlines in the media. But most of those with reduced longevity also had substance abuse and/or personality disorders, which are themselves markers for a shorter lifespan.

The most striking change in current practice is that physicians are now prescribing stimulants much more often to adults, not just to children with problems in school.

I blame physicians, both primary care providers and psychiatrists, for diagnosing and prescribing these agents too freely. We do not know if they have problematic effects if taken for decades. It should also be known, but is not, that cognitive behavioral therapy has research support for ADHD (Young et al., 2020). A decision to prescribe nonpsychotic patients with medication for years to come should not be taken lightly.

2.9 Overdiagnosis of Autism Spectrum Disorder

Autism spectrum disorder (ASD) presents similar problems for overdiagnosis (Fombonne, 2023). In this case, there is no pharmacological treatment driving diagnosis, but ASD can be embraced as an explanation for social awkwardness. Recently, the concept of a spectrum of psychopathology has encouraged this diagnosis by allowing it to be made in cases with fewer features of the disorder (O'Sullivan, 2025).

Originally there were two types in the DSM – classical autism (associated with major cognitive defects) and Asperger's syndrome (in which patients are much more functional). Even if the decision in DSM-5 to combine these clinical presentations was justified, the introduction of a dimensional "spectrum" opens the door to diagnostic inflation. Autism is all too often applied to anyone with excess social anxiety. While ASD has no specific treatment, patients and families ask for this diagnosis because it supports specialized forms of education for disabled children.

2.10 Overdiagnosis of Depression

Few diagnoses in psychiatry are as common as depression. But its clinical picture is heterogeneous. Once again, following the manual can point us in the wrong direction.

Since DSM-III was published, psychiatrists have assumed that "major depression" is one illness that only varies in severity. But in DSM-I and DSM-II, it was two disorders. The first was "reactive depression," describing a pathological response to loss. The second was a severe condition called "psychotic depression." This basis for this separation was problematic, since severe depression can be triggered by a loss and does not necessarily involve psychotic symptoms. But that does not prove that major depression describes forms of a single disorder (Lynall and McIntosh, 2023). DSM-5-TR does allow for modifiers of this diagnosis (recurrent, psychotic, melancholic), but are not always used in practice.

Unfortunately, under the influence of a group of experts who believed that *all* depressed patients should be treated with antidepressants, DSM-III adopted a unitary model of major depression. (There was never a category of minor depression). But if depressed mood is just a symptom, like fever or inflammation, it is no wonder that only about half of patients receiving these medications go into remission (see Chapter 5).

Another problem is that depression, at least in the DSM system, no longer has a context. Previous editions had allowed for a *grief exclusion*, instructed clinicians to withhold a diagnosis after a major loss such as the death of a loved one. The rationale was that grief can develop into a clinical depression that needs treatment (Kendler et al., 2008). This decision was criticized by Wakefield (2007) as an unjustified medicalization of normal sadness and the human condition. As he pointed out, grief is a process that can last for many months if not years. This is why DSM-5-TR allows for a diagnosis of prolonged grief disorder (Killikelly et al., 2025). But it is not established how long normal grief should last.

The Australian psychiatrist Gordon Parker (2000) has published many papers on the heterogeneity of depression. Here is what he wrote 20 years ago (Parker, 2005, p. 473):

> [T]he "final common pathway" model, articulated in the early 1970s, helped to cement psychiatric classification in subsequent DSM and ICD revisions into a unitarian framework, leading to a relatively sterile period of depression research. Clinically described depressive typologies were obscured rather than refined by appropriate modeling paradigms. A contrasting, empirically based hierarchical model, driven by disorder-specific clinical manifestations such as psychotic features and observable psychomotor disturbance, is proposed as a paradigm for distinguishing psychotic, melancholic, and non-melancholic classes of depression, while a spectrum model is favored for distinguishing the principal non-melancholic subclasses.

Sad to say, neither DSM nor ICD have taken Parker's recommendations to heart. The result is that psychiatry has medicalized sadness and that depressed patients are not being offered a choice between treatment options.

Depression is being overdiagnosed. The media, backed by researchers, have some-times worried readers by claiming that the prevalence of common mental disorders (depression and anxiety) is going up. However, it is not clear whether diagnoses have increased as more clinicians are looking to make them, or whether more patients are asking for help with milder symptoms (Baxter et al., 2014).

One might also conclude that life is just not that happy, and that most people will suffer from periods of sadness. However, there is evidence for an increase among adolescent girls, which some social psychologists date to the rise of social media (Twenge, 2023). Ormel et al. (2022) note, as a paradox, that in spite of greater availability of treatment for depression, its prevalence has not gone down. That suggests that psychiatry has exaggerated the efficacy of its treatments.

2.11 Overdiagnosis of PTSD

The diagnosis of post-traumatic stress disorder (PTSD) follows from the view, discussed previously, that adverse life events can, by themselves, cause mental disorders. Making this diagnosis can also lead to offering what has been called "trauma-informed" psycho-therapy. Although other overdiagnoses are based on biological theories, PTSD is rooted in sympathy for the victims of traumatic life events. The clinical picture of this disorder is dominated by flashbacks, nightmares, and the avoidance of environmental "triggers."

As discussed earlier, most people exposed to trauma, even when severe, never develop PTSD, and the overall prevalence after exposure to a stressor is 5–10% (McNally, 2003; Paris, 2023c). PTSD is more common in women, and rape is the most likely adverse event to lead to symptoms, affecting 20% of those exposed (Scott et al., 2018).

But those who develop PTSD symptoms have other risk factors that are more important: higher levels of trait neuroticism, as well as either a personal and/or a family history of mental disorder. PTSD is an excellent example of a diagnosis that does not have a simple cause but arises from complex pathways that are biopsychosocial.

So why do some patients *want* to have PTSD? One reason is that this diagnosis validates suffering and the right to be angry about mistreatment. Also, PTSD is popular because it provides a simple explanation for complex problems, and one that shifts the blame from oneself to other people. Still another reason is that services can be more available if you have this disorder, as is the case for clients of the Veterans

Administration in the USA. I have practiced in Canada, where psychiatric care is insured by governments, but psychotherapy outside of hospitals is not. Even so, my province (Quebec) has a program that pays for extended psychotherapy by a psychologist if a patient has a trauma history (with or without a formal diagnosis of PTSD).

It has long been known that war veterans can develop PTSD symptoms, but those affected are still in the minority. Today, more clinical attention is given to trauma in civilian life. The overall prevalence after any exposure to adverse life events shows that most people do not develop the disorder. If most people are resilient, even to the worst kind of trauma, there must be factors other than exposure in the risk for PTSD. A large body of evidence supports the conclusion that resilience is the most common response to life stressors (Paris, 2023c).

Even so, PTSD can be a useful diagnosis, and a number of therapies for this syndrome are known to be effective, even though none is superior to any other (McLean et al., 2022). However, I see PTSD being used to describe patients who have only had a difficult childhood, often with what might better be called emotional neglect, without discrete traumatic experiences. The concept of trauma has been subject to "construct creep" (Jones and McNally, 2022), and is being overused for the large number of patients whose upbringing leaves much to be desired.

Another diagnosis that has been adopted rapidly in recent years is *complex PTSD* (Paris, 2023c). This condition is mentioned in the ICD-11, but not in the DSM-5. Its description in the ICD manual overlaps with several features of borderline personality disorder (BPD). It also includes several characteristic features of PTSD (reexperiencing, avoidance, and hypervigilance), but adds on *emotional dysregulation, interpersonal difficulties, interpersonal difficulties*, and *a negative self-concept*. These additional features are typical of a personality disorder. PTSD has a 25–30% comorbidity with BPD (Pagura et al., 2010). But in my view, research does not support the implication that PDs are mainly caused by trauma and can be a form of PTSD (Paris, 2023c); rather, it is one of several risk factors that can lead to this outcome. DSM-5 did not go along with a diagnosis of complex PTSD, only allowing for a severe form of PTSD itself.

Complex PTSD has been popular, even in North America where the ICD system is not often used. The reason is the same as that for PTSD itself, in that it attributes complex pathology to the direct effects of adverse experiences, consistent with the overvaluation of trauma that afflicts modern psychiatry. This diagnosis seems to explain psychopathology, but it fails to distinguish correlation from causation.

2.12 Overdiagnosis and Self-Diagnosis

The internet is a technology that has been helpful for almost everyone. But patients are now using it for self-diagnosis. They can find information about the criteria for mental disorders online (if they find the right site – given that search engines rank websites by popularity, not by reliability).

The problem is that when diagnostic criteria are easily available on the web, patients can diagnose themselves prior to consulting a physician, and to arrive convinced of their own conclusions. They may come to consultations asking for a specific treatment, usually medication. I can understand these requests, since like the clinicians who evaluate them, patients are looking for answers. And since most psychiatrists these days restrict their practice to prescriptions, they are all too ready to offer medications to people with common problems that may not meet criteria for a diagnosis of a mental disorder. Thus, both parties may be attracted to conditions that can be self-diagnosed.

2.13 Prospects for the Future of Classification in Mental Disorders

Neuroscience has not been able to keep its promises to psychiatry. The reason is that the diagnoses we use, particularly the 350 or so in the DSM manual, are not real categories of illness, but syndromes. As long as that is the case, classifying mental disorders by observable symptoms will be limited by the absence of a guiding theory. Until we find biomarkers, further revisions in diagnostic manuals can be based only on guesses and opinions.

Answer to Unanswered Question #2

Given that we do not know the causes of most mental disorders, classifying them remains problematic. The DSM and ICD systems are at best tools for provisional use. Dimensional alternatives can add more information, but are also not based on etiology. Meanwhile, a number of the categories the manuals list are being faddishly overdiagnosed.

Biopsychosocial

Unanswered Question #3: Can adherence to a biopsychosocial model of mental disorders inform clinical practice?

3.1 The Biopsychosocial Model

As Chapters 1 and 2 have shown, to understand and classify mental disorders, we will need major advances in brain science to allow us to make diagnoses based on causes rather than symptoms. However, that is only part of the story. A neuroscience-based model would be most useful for the disorders that have the largest component of heritability, that is, psychoses and severe mood disorders. In most of the patients psychiatrists see, psychosocial factors are at least as important. Unfortunately, those who defend the role of the environment in psychopathology may fail to take proper account of the role played by heritable factors, especially temperament and personality traits. These relationships will be examined in Chapter 4.

No single risk factor accounts for the development of mental illnesses or can be used in a scientific classification. We need a model that is multivariate and interactive. The most useful theory, proposed nearly half a century ago, attempted to do just that.

George Engel was an internist interested in psychosomatic medicine, who was dissatisfied with the biomedical model of human diseases. He noted strong evidence from health psychology research that psychosocial risk factors play an important role in many medical illnesses. This led him to write a paper (Engel, 1977) advocating a biopsychosocial (BPS) model that was broader, more holistic, and that could be used by physicians to provide better care for patients.

Engel (1980) then extended his model to show how it could be applied to psychiatry. This was an obvious application, but its timing was in part a response to a paradigm shift, as more psychiatrists began to embrace a biomedical model. As DSM-III was about to be published, Engel aimed to counter this narrowly biological approach to mental illness. He also wanted to avoid the exclusively psychological models that dominated the practice of psychotherapy but take little account of individual differences in environmental sensitivity. For Engel, medicine treats people, not puzzles in neuroscience or in reexperiencing the drama of past traumas.

Most psychiatrists today, at least in principle, see themselves as guided by Engel's approach. A book of 23 chapters was published a few years ago, and it nicely covers the field (Savulescu et al., 2020). But the BPS model is not without its critics. Some see it as vague or nonspecific (Ghaemi, 2011). Let us therefore consider what the model is and what it is not.

It is true that the BPS does not tell you precisely how biological and psychosocial factors interact, or how they contribute to specific clinical pictures. That is due to our lack of a detailed understanding of how the brain processes life experiences (Frances, 2014). Instead, the model aims to counter biases that are based on oversimplified theories that fail to take complexity into account. It is more like a globe than a detailed map.

The problem with the biomedical model is that it only pays lip service to the role of the environment and might better be termed a "bio-bio-bio model" (Whitley, 2014). Today many clinicians and researchers see mental disorders as nothing but defects in neuronal wiring or neurotransmission.

As we have seen, leaders such as the former director of the National Institute of Mental Health (NIMH) have attempted to redefine psychiatry as a clinical application of neuroscience. Yet considering the complexity of such a task, research thus far has not been impressive. If the mind is an emergent property of the brain, accounting for psychopathology at a neuronal level is unlikely to succeed (Bolton, 2023).

For much the same reason, environmental cannot be understood without considering how biological variations determine how the brain processes them. Moreover, everyone has unique life experiences that are "unshared" and not accounted for by their family environment. Monozygotic twins are not born entirely identical, and epigenetic changes in the genome can arise from life experience (Fitz-James and Cavalli, 2022; Holliday, 2006).

The BPS model can be considered as an elaboration of older diathesis-stress models (Rende and Plomin, 1992). It is not a predictive theory, but a broad framework for understanding mental illness. Its model supports a humanistic practice that focuses on the whole person.

The BPS model also does not offer a quantitative scale that can be applied in research. It does not support simply adding up multiple risk and protective factors but hypothesizes interactions between them in development. Proving that this is so requires research in large samples, using valid measures of psychosocial factors, and then carrying out longitudinal follow-ups. That is why data remains relatively scarce on the clinical application of the model. We need more genetically informed studies that follow children into adulthood.

Finally, a BPS model assessing multiple risk and protective factors helps account for the ubiquity of resilience. The fact that most people are not permanently affected by traumatic events is consistent with the concept that we have a *psychological immune system* that promotes resilience to stressors (Gilbert, 1995; Rosenzweig, 2016). Thus, we are not passive recipients of adverse life events but have evolved systems to detoxify them (Rutter, 2013). That is why resilience is so ubiquitous (Bonanno, 2021).

Psychiatry requires an openness to multiple causation (Kendler, 2005). That is also the view of Bolton (2008), a psychologist and philosopher who has written about the problems of classifying mental disorders. In a recent book, Bolton and Gillett (2019) argued that the BPS model and multiple causation make room for *agency* in the study of brain and behavior. Much the same point has been made by neuroscientists who consider agency and free will to be an evolutionary adaptation (e.g., Mitchell, 2023). Similarly, Kendler (2019) has pointed out the need for "multilevel" studies of psychopathology. The deficiency of the biomedical model is that it treats the mind as a machine without agency.

3.2 How Do Biology and Psychology Interact?

Some brain functions are strongly heritable; They have to be to control processes that are necessary for survival (Smoller, 2017). The large size of the human brain reflects a capacity to process life experiences and to manage social interactions, that is, the "social brain" (Dunbar, 2009). Brain development is a complex process, and it has a random component related to neural migration prior to birth and over the course of childhood (Mitchell, 2018, 2023).

In this perspective, one can see why biology and psychology are closely intertwined. Our environment modifies and shapes the brain. That may be one reason why psychotherapy, which helps patients to process life experiences in a better way, is at least as effective as medication in the management of common mental disorders (Cuijpers et al., 2020).

One intensively studied interactive mechanism is *epigenetics* (Holliday, 2006). Life experiences can modify the genome by activating or silencing its packaging (made of methyl groups or histones). These changes can sometimes be passed on over several generations. For example, children who were in their mother's womb during the Dutch famine of 1945 were later found to be more at risk for obesity, diabetes, and schizophrenia; these changes in methylation of the genome were also seen in their children and grandchildren (Lumey, 2016). But while epigenetics is a factor in the complex pathways to psychopathology, its specific mechanisms have not yet been identified.

3.3 Complexity, Reductionism, and Emergence

The human brain is a prime example of a complex system (Ladyman et al., 2013). Its development is marked by multiple interactions whose outcomes are nonlinear, not fully predictable, and that can only be measured as probabilities. That is another reason why studying the mind on a strictly neural level is not the best way to advance brain science. Let us examine why the neuroscience research community has favored that approach.

Reductionism, that is, breaking down complex phenomena into their components, has been a winning strategy in many scientific domains. But complex systems cannot be fully explained in that way. Instead, they have *emergent* properties that could not have been predicted by observations on a simpler level (Byrne and Callaghan, 2022). We need to embrace this complexity, allowing for the emergence of phenomena that are not apparent when reduced to single variables with linear relationships (Öngür and Paulus, 2025).

In psychiatry, a reductionistic approach to psychopathology is unlikely to succeed and needs to be replaced with studies on multiple levels. Thus, we cannot hope to explain human behavior at the level of neurons unless we also take data from the social sciences into account.

A philosopher of psychiatry (Gold, 2009, p. 511) came to similar conclusions:

> What skepticism about reduction does imply is that an understanding of mental illness and its treatment is unlikely to come solely from biology. As plausible as it is that neuroscience is necessary to psychiatry, it is equally plausible that various branches of psychology, sociology, anthropology, and other disciplines will be equally or more important.

A similar perspective comes from a leading researcher in psychiatric genetics who has published widely on the philosophy of psychiatry. Kendler (2005, p. 437) concluded:

> Multilevel models, especially those including mental and social explanatory perspectives, are typically rejected (sometimes with the epithet of being non-scientific or "soft-headed") or accepted only with the caveat that all the "real" causal effects occur at the level of basic biology. This position might be seen as a logical consequence of the rejection of Cartesian dualism. After all, if we agree that there are no mental processes that are independent of brain function, then should not all the causes of psychiatric disorders be reduced to brain processes? Although this reductionist perspective is understandable in sociological terms as a reaction to prior radical mentalistic programs within psychiatry (e.g., some forms of dynamic psychiatry) and is appealing because of the ease with which it fits into a medical model, this approach is too narrow to encompass the range of causal processes that are operative in psychiatric disorders.

3.4 Clinical Implications of the BPS Model

The BPS model can be applied to many diseases in medicine, especially chronic illnesses. The number of published articles that use this model has increased in recent years (Wade and Halligan, 2017). But thus far, the main impact of BPS has been in psychiatry.

The great majority of mental disorders can be best understood in this model. Let us now, very briefly, examine what we know.

3.4.1 Psychoses

Schizophrenia has a large heritable component. The genome-wide association studies (GWAS) yield polygenic risk scores from several hundred sites that accounts for up to 80% of the total variance (Legge et al., 2021). Yet even in disorders that carry a heavy genetic load, there is a role for psychosocial stressors. For example, schizophrenia is more likely to develop under conditions of "social defeat" (Selten and Cantor-Graae, 2007). Long-term use of cannabis is also a risk factor. But these pathways are most likely to affect those who already have a genetic predisposition to the disorder. In that way, schizophrenia is most like chronic illnesses in medicine.

Bipolar-I disorder is also highly heritable, and its clinical picture frequently includes periods of psychosis during manic episodes. There is some evidence that childhood adversity can be an additional risk factor (Rowland and Marwaha, 2018). Bipolar-II is a less severe disorder, marked by hypomania. However, its boundaries are fuzzy, and this diagnosis remains controversial (Malhi et al., 2019). Moreover, differential diagnosis of bipolarity with personality disorders can be difficult, especially when mood swings are a prominent feature (Paris, 2009a). Psychosocial risk factors may play a role in both forms of bipolarity but are not specific to the diagnosis (Marangoni et al., 2016). Like most forms of psychopathology, bipolarity arises from heritable risks that are activated by life stressors.

3.4.2 Mood and Anxiety Disorders

Major depression is a heterogenous group of symptoms that has long been considered to be a single disorder that can be more or less severe. Thus, while mood disorders tend to be more frequent when people suffer a loss, extended periods of normal grief can be confused with depression (Wakefield, 2013). Depressions that have "melancholic" features may lack obvious precursors (Parker, 2005), but even milder depressions reflect some degree of biological vulnerability (Su et al., 2024).

Flint and Kendler (2014) reviewed the research literature on the role of genes, and found support for the view, as argued by others (Parker, 2000), that "major depression" is not a single disorder, but a heterogeneous group. Moreover, genetic markers, even when based on GWAS data, did not explain these variations. The problem is with the definition of major depression itself, which masks this heterogeneity. As Flint and Kendler conclude (2014, p. 497):

> As might have been predicted from a set of criteria chosen on the basis of clinical judgment rather than psychometric properties or validation from biological features, the nine *DSM* symptomatic criteria for MD do not appear to represent a single underlying genetic factor.

Flint and Kendler go on to observe that there is strong evidence showing that people who develop depression have an increased sensitivity to environmental stressors. In other words, these patients are high in neuroticism. This is a domain of personality that is most often linked with mental disorders (Widiger and Oltmanns, 2017). That trait may also be a basis of gene-environment interactions that best account for the emergence of depressive episodes. That is why understanding depression requires a biopsychosocial model. What it does not require is a knee-jerk diagnosis of major depression, followed in almost every case by prescriptions that may not be helpful.

Anxiety disorders – which include panic, generalized anxiety, and social anxiety – are very common, and can be comorbid with each other as well as with depression (Chen, 2022). Anxiety usually begins in childhood and has a strong relation to temperament, but it can be exacerbated by adverse life events (Newman et al., 2013).

3.4.3 Substance Use Disorders

Substance use requires access to a substance, as shown by wide variations in prevalence around the world, largely related to culture (Mackinnon et al., 2017). But the tendency either to become addicted or to be a problematic user is strongly heritable, and the most severe cases often begin in adolescence (Deak and Johnson, 2021). This is a complex but highly prevalent group of disorders that require a biopsychosocial theory (MacKillop and Ray, 2017).

3.4.4 Eating Disorders

This group (anorexia nervosa, bulimia, and binge eating) is also a prime candidate for biopsychosocial modeling. These conditions are related to heritable traits (Bulik et al., 2022). But their psychosocial roots are even stronger (Smolak and Levine, 2015), as shown in the role of social contagion in increased prevalence. As many clinical phenomena can increase or decrease rapidly over time, Shorter (1992) has described these changes as a common source of psychopathology drawing from a "symptom pool."

3.4.5 Post-Traumatic Stress Disorder

Even in disorders triggered by a toxic environment, biology plays a role. As discussed in Chapter 2, the best example is PTSD (Calhoun et al., 2022), rooted in high levels of trait neuroticism that undermine resilience, rather like an alarm system that cannot be turned off. I have written a book about gene-environment interactions on PTSD (Paris, 2023c), emphasizing how research shows that these symptoms are most likely to appear in those with neurotic traits.

3.4.6 Personality Disorders

For a particularly clear-cut application of the BPS Model, let us look at personality disorder (PD), the focus of my own research (Paris, 2015a, 2022b). These symptomatically complex conditions are derived from heritable trait profiles, stressful life circumstances, and a lack of social support. Their complexity has made them difficult to classify, but PDs cannot be understood at the level of neurons. We will return to these disorders in Chapter 4.

3.5 Putting the Pieces of Psychopathology Back Together

Every year since 1948, the BBC has broadcast (and now podcasts) a series of talks called the Reith Lectures. Its aim is to advance public understanding about issues of contemporary interest. In 2024, the Reith lectures were given for the first time by a psychiatrist.

Gwen Adshead, a British forensic specialist, argued that many if not most violent behaviors, including homicide, can be successfully treated with psychotherapy. One of the four Reith lectures was devoted to the role of childhood trauma in violent behaviors in adults. Adshead acknowledged that it is rare for survivors of trauma to become criminals, and that early adversity is only one of many risk factors leaning to that outcome. However, she failed to mention that a good deal of evidence shows that antisocial behaviors also have a heritable component.

Consider, for example, the Dunedin study in New Zealand that has been following a birth cohort from 1972 to 1973 of 1,037 children who are now in their fifties (Poulton et al., 2023). This group was the source of a study that I criticized in Chapter 1 for confining itself to the effects of single genes. But we now have data from this cohort, as well as another (the E-Risk study from the UK), that used GWAS (Wertz et al., 2018). What these authors found (p. 791) was:

> Polygenic risk manifested during primary schooling in lower cognitive abilities, lower self-control, academic difficulties, and truancy, and it was associated with a life-course-persistent pattern of antisocial behavior that onsets in childhood and persists
> into adulthood.

However, the authors noted that the effect size of polygenic risk scores was small relative to other predictors (e.g., parental antisocial behavior, cognitive ability). While genetic risk cannot be the main explanation for violence, for an expert giving the Reith lectures not to even mention its heritability is a good example of the biases that psychotherapists all too often hold. The most evidence-based view is that trauma is most pathogenic for those who already have emotions prone to dysregulation.

I was also surprised to hear Adshead express puzzlement at the fact that the vast majority of violent crimes are committed by men. She went on to wonder if women are more resilient to stressors (which is certainly not the case). Having a Y chromosome, while not a direct cause, is by far the strongest risk for violent behaviors of all kinds (Archer, 2022). Being male is the strongest risk factor for death by suicide, in which men typically use violent methods. All these differences are mediated by testosterone levels, which are of course much higher in males.

It is also simplistic to focus on genetic risk factors, which some assume can fully explain the onset of mental illness. Even when using GWAS, which is a more sophisticated point of view than used in earlier genetic research, the solution to resolving these complexities remains obscure.

I have seen tens of thousands of patients over the course of a long career. I do not claim that my clinical experience is as valid as systematic research. But I applied the biopsychosocial model every day over several decades. When patients would ask me to explain why they were ill, I would usually say something like this: "You have always been unusually sensitive when bad things happen to you, and you have had to deal with several of them." But that response reflects the fact that most of my patients have had diagnoses of personality disorders, not psychoses or severe mood disorders.

Attempts at reducing all forms of psychopathology to neural connections is not just a problem in theory. The overuse of biomedical models that lies behind clinical management consisting of a prescription and little else. While skilled clinicians can assess patients in 30 minutes, 15 minutes is just not enough. In summary, both the medicalization of psychiatry and the narrow psychological models that have dominated clinical psychology lead to impoverished choices.

3.6 Prospects for the Biopsychosocial Model

Kenneth Kendler is a prolific American professor of psychiatry with one of the highest citation indexes. In an eloquent defense of the BPS model, Kendler and Gygnell (2020, p. 25) concluded:

> [T]he non-additive relationship between risk factors at different causal levels provides reasons to resist hard reductionist models of psychiatric disorders. Similarly, it argues that psychiatry should resist attempts to base classification schemes on a hard medical model. Instead, psychiatry should embrace the fuzzy and complex causal picture that research suggests reflects the true nature of mental illness.

In other words, psychiatry has fundamental differences from other domains of medicine. It is not a subdiscipline of neurology. That is not to claim that medicine as a whole does not need a BPS model; it does. But the relative importance of psychosocial risk factors is greater in many mental disorders. That is also why psychiatry, which is about the mind, is not the same thing as neurology. (That does not imply a philosophical dualism, but reflects how clinicians practice, and the questions they ask their patients.) If we try to turn psychiatry into an application of neuroscience, we cannot do justice to what other domains of research tell us. We will also continue overdiagnosing and overprescribing, without understanding the complex world of psychopathology.

This brings us to the idea of biopsychosocial treatment methods. Many of our patients need both pharmacological and psychotherapeutic interventions. The use of this combination, particular to good psychiatric practice, is more likely to lead to a remission of mental symptoms.

Answer to Unanswered Question #3
Psychiatry needs to apply a biopsychosocial model and give it more than lip service in understanding and treating psychopathology. This means we should blame neither genes nor neural connections or families for mental illness. The BPS model combines all these risk factors into a single theory and accounts for the complexity of these disorders in treatment.

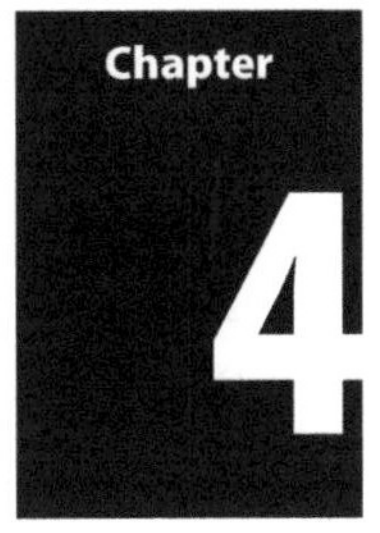

Chapter 4

Personality, Traits, and Personality Disorders

Unanswered Question #4: Do psychiatrists need to stop centering their practice on symptoms, and allow a more central role for personality traits?

4.1 Defining and Classifying Personality

Psychiatric diagnoses are based on clinical observation and patient reports. Most of our treatments focus on symptoms. Clinicians do a good job in providing relief from symptoms but are less successful at modifying the traits that make patients vulnerable. Doing so requires a deeper understanding of how the brain works, and how people respond to environmental challenges. As of now, we are in an equivalent position to the practice of medicine in the past: reducing symptoms but lacking a theory that would allow us to target underlying biological mechanisms.

The term *endophenotype* refers to heritable variations that are intermediate between biology and clinical symptoms (Gottesman and Gould, 2003). We can only rarely identify these markers. For example, some patients with schizophrenia have abnormal eye movements that reflect abnormal functioning of the frontal cortex (Wolf et al., 2021). But that endophenotype lacks specificity. Only about half of patients with the disorder have the biomarker, which in any case does not tell us what precisely is wrong in the brain. Up to now, while researchers have been actively searching for endophenotypes for mental illness, hardly any have been identified.

There are also broader features at a more theoretical level that are not clinically apparent but are risk factors for mental disorders of all kinds. A *psychopathology* or *p-factor* is common to a very wide range of diagnoses (Caspi et al., 2014). But this measure cannot predict who will and who will not develop any specific form of psychopathology.

A better bet would be to measure *personality* traits. In psychology, these profiles describe enduring characteristics and behavior that shape unique adjustments to life's challenges (Paris, 2023a). People have notable individual differences in the way they think, feel, and behave. These traits remain fairly consistent over time, but change to some extent with maturity (Widiger, 2015).

We know a good deal about the nature of personality. The most convincing data, discussed in Chapter 1, comes from behavior genetics (Jang, 2005). Thus, twin studies show that *all* personality traits have a heritable component that accounts for close to half the outcome variance in populations. But the environmental component in personality is largely "unshared," that is, not affected to any great extent by growing up in a particular family. Since these effects are not "shared," siblings can be as different in traits as perfect strangers.

This conclusion surprised psychotherapists who had always assumed that childhood experiences profoundly shape adult functioning. In spite of decades of confirming behavior genetic data, some clinicians either refuse to believe what research has shown or do their best to minimize these findings. But they may not surprise parents who observe how different each of their children are from each other. That observation contradicts theories that search for childhood life events to explain why patients have difficulty as adults. It does not mean that life events have no effects, but that most responses to adversity occur in people with an increased sensitivity to their environment.

Behavioral genetic findings do not imply that biological vulnerability by itself can explain why people develop mental disorders. Applying a biopsychosocial model will be needed to conduct research showing how heritable traits and adverse experiences interact to increase the risk for pathological outcomes.

4.2 The Five Factor Model of Personality

Over the last century, there have been many proposals for the best way to classify personality traits. The most extensive research has supported high reliability and validity for the *Five Factor Model* (FFM; Widiger, 2015). This system describes five broad trait domains, each of which can be adaptive or maladaptive, depending on the nature of environmental challenges. Each of the five factors can then be divided into six *facets* (although facets are rarely used in clinical work).

Personality domains emerge from responses to self-report questionnaires that can then be grouped by factor analysis into the "Big Five": *extraversion, neuroticism, openness to experience, agreeableness,* and *conscientiousness.* (If you have trouble remembering them, you can use the acronym "OCEAN.")

Extraversion vs. Introversion describes how much people need to connect (or not) with others in social networks and close relationships. Extraverts prefer to be around others and to interact with them. Introverts have less need for intimacy and spend much of their time on interests that do not require social interaction.

Neuroticism vs. Emotional Stability describes the strength of negative and/or dysregulated emotions when facing stressful life events. High neuroticism is associated with many mental disorders that lead people to see psychiatrists or other therapists (Widiger and Oltmanns, 2017). At the other end of this spectrum, emotional stability is less associated with psychopathology but can sometimes risk failure to perceive real threats.

Agreeableness vs. Antagonism describes the extent to which people need to please others or to oppose them. Antagonism is a problematic trait, as it interferes with establishing and maintaining relationships. High agreeableness is usually positive, but can be associated with naiveté in social life and to a vulnerability to manipulation.

Conscientiousness vs. Impulsivity describes whether people persist in carry out tasks in life or act on impulse. Being conscientious is usually a positive trait, strongly associated with better health and success in life. But at an extreme, it can turn into perfectionism and be associated with a personality disorder. Impulsivity is associated with a high risk for mental disorders, as this trait gets people into conflicts that eventually lead to symptoms.

Openness to Experience vs. Closed to Experience describes whether people are interested or uninterested in new ideas. This trait lacks a strong relationship to any form of psychopathology.

The FFM model is based on the factor analysis of responses to self-report questionnaires. That statistical technique defines the five factors based on the intercorrelation of these responses. One might wonder whether people can accurately describe their own personalities. Almost all of us have blind spots about our deficiencies, and some prefer to blame others for their problems. This bias has been described as a "fundamental attribution error" (Ross, 2018), in which people explain their own mistakes by circumstance, and overemphasize personality traits as the cause of mistakes made by others. But by and large, self-report data about traits on the FFM and similar models can be confirmed by interview data (Helle et al., 2017), and by their ability to predict outcomes such as longevity, illness, and mental disorders (Widiger, 2015).

Here it may be useful to comment on *narcissism*, a personality trait that has launched a thousand books. High narcissism, associated with attention seeking and grandiosity, is not part of the FFM, but has its own scales for measurement. Narcissists do not often come for help, since they see their own personality as positive, and usually blame others for any problems.

While most psychiatrists are not familiar with the FFM, it is easy to learn, as it uses plain language instead of jargon. In view of the large body of research on the FFM, I have wondered why this system was not adopted by either the ICD or the DSM manuals – instead of developing new systems of their own. Some clinicians view this system, developed in community populations, as not doing full justice to severe psychopathology. Even so, alternatives to the FFM can be used to diagnose personality disorders. (See discussion of ICD-11 and the Alternative Model for Personality Disorders in Sections 4.3 and 4.4, respectively). Both use four of the five factors. To some extent, the FFM can also explain why people develop specific mental disorders. Its profiles track both inner states of mind and dysfunctional patterns of behavior.

Overall, the best predictor of dysfunction in life is high neuroticism (Widiger and Oltmanns, 2017). This trait is associated with higher levels of anxiety, depression, and personality disorders. Its ubiquity is also consistent with current trends in clinical psychology that highlight emotion dysregulation as a target for therapy in many categories of mental disorder.

Each personality profile can be adaptive in the right environment. Even neuroticism has a purpose in that it constitutes an early alert system to identify environmental threats. But there are times when traits work against us rather than for us. Many problems can be seen as amplifications of traits by adverse life experiences. One can also observe a vicious circle in which traits interfere with functioning, leading to further amplification.

4.3 Personality and Personality Disorders

We all have a personality. But clinicians should only diagnose a *personality disorder* (PD) when traits are clearly dysfunctional. The overall definition of a PD in ICD-11 (World Health Organization, 2018) is "a disturbance in self and interpersonal functioning that is enduring and manifests as maladaptive patterns of behavior, cognition, and emotional experience. The disturbances must be present for at least two years." The DSM-5-TR definition (American Psychiatric Association, 2022) is similar: "[A] long-term pattern of behavior and inner experiences that significantly differs from what is expected in a person's culture. These patterns are inflexible and consistent across situations and can lead to distress or impairment."

Personality disorders have always been controversial. Some psychiatrists rarely diagnose them, at least on a regular basis, preferring to focus on the depression and anxiety that often accompany a PD. But it is a mistake to focus on distress without considering what kind of person is distressed. As the physician William Osler (https://litfl.com/eponymictionary/oslerisms/) is quoted as having said: "[T]he good physician treats the disease; the great physician treats the patient who has the disease."

What makes the definition and classification of personality disorders difficult is a fuzzy boundary with normal variations. Some clinicians worry that people receive these diagnoses just because they are different. Actually, the problem of establishing a boundary between normality and psychopathology applies to many disorders in the manual (Frances, 2013). When explaining the concept of PD to patients (who may ask me if they have a "bad" personality), I explain that these diagnoses describe people whose problems in relationships and career plans run into serious obstacles over time in achieving life goals.

Thus, we should reserve PD diagnoses to cases in which trait profiles are extreme and in which functioning is seriously compromised. And when trait profiles are quantitative rather than qualitative, they can also be used to measure personality in nonclinical populations. Normal variations in traits are more related to personality structure than to diagnoses of mental disorders (Hyman, 2021).

4.4 Alternative Model for Personality Disorders

The editors of DSM-5 asked their work group on personality disorders to come up with a dimensional measure for PDs that would eventually be a test case for expanding quantitative diagnoses to all mental disorders. This system is now known as the *Alternative Model for Personality Disorders* (AMPD). It is a "hybrid" model in which the total number of PD categories is reduced from 10 to 6, while those that remain are rooted in trait profiles. The AMPD does not assume that PD categories are "natural kinds" in the same way as medical diagnoses.

In 2013, after much discussion, the AMPD was not fully approved, as further data was required to support a radical change. Instead, it was placed in Section III of the DSM-5 (for diagnoses requiring more research). But the AMPD may still make it into the main part of the DSM, perhaps in DSM-6, or in a revised version of the AMPD that is currently under review by a committee. This system combines many of the advantages of dimensional scoring of traits, without completely removing familiar and clinically important diagnoses (such as BPD).

AMPD diagnoses are made in two steps (Hopwood, 2019). First is Criterion A, in which one must determine if there is a significant dysfunction in self and identity, along with problems in interpersonal relationships. A questionnaire can be used to measure this criterion, the Personality Inventory for DSM-5 (PID-5; Al-Dajani et al., 2016). The second step is Criterion B, which describes a set of trait profiles associated with six categories of PD – schizotypal, antisocial, borderline, narcissistic, avoidant, and obsessive-compulsive disorders.

One advantage of using this system is that it does not lose information by encasing data in categories that do not quite fit. Another is that it avoids the confusion created by the tendency of patients to meet criteria for more than one category, or to fall within the vast realm of "PD unspecified" (Zimmerman et al., 2005).

The AMPD would be a major change. PDs have long been classified, both in ICD and DSM, as a group of categorical diagnoses. But only two of the current DSM categories have a large body of empirical research to support their validity. The first is what DSM-5-TR calls *antisocial PD* (*dissocial PD* in ICD-10). These categories, along with a more severe form called *psychopathy*, are of importance to forensic psychiatry.

The second, *borderline* PD – which describes a pattern of mood instability, impulsivity, and problematic relationships – has been intensively researched over the last half century. Its features also include suicidal behaviors and self-harm (Zimmerman et al., 2005).

There have now been thousands of published papers on BPD, and this disorder has been the focus of my own career. I began by being intrigued by the problem of chronic suicidality, and then, with the help of colleagues, retrained myself as a researcher. Later, applying the principles of specialized psychotherapies developed for BPD, I founded a network of clinics devoted to managing this challenging population.

4.5 The ICD-11 Model of Personality Disorders

The ICD-11 (World Health Organization, 2018) aimed to eliminate *all* PD categories, and to replace them with five dimensions of personality (whether normal or abnormal) that can be quantitatively scored: *negative affectivity, dissociality, anankastia, detachment,* and *disinhibition.* These factors closely resemble four factors in the FFM. Thus, negative affectivity tracks neuroticism, detachment tracks low extraversion, dissociality tracks low agreeableness, disinhibition tracks low conscientiousness, while anankastia tracks high conscientiousness.

The original ICD-11 proposal met with pushback from researchers in Europe and North America who had spent decades studying BPD (Herpertz et al., 2017). There were several reasons for opposition to eliminating that diagnosis. First, BPD is by far the most researched of any PD. It is also unusually difficult to manage, as chronic suicidality challenges and frightens clinicians. Moreover, complexity arises because BPD has both internalizing and externalizing clinical features, making it more difficult to dimensionalize (Eaton et al., 2011). However, the diagnosis of BPD is gradually becoming more acceptable to clinicians as the disorder is now known to remit with time, and to respond to specific psychological treatments.

The final decision for ICD-11 was a compromise, in which clinicians are still allowed to identify a *borderline pattern*, whose description is much the same as the one in DSM-5-TR (Simonsen and Paris, 2025). Peter Tyrer, who headed the ICD-11 committee on PDs, and who has been a long-term critic of the BPD construct, objected to this outcome (Mulder and Tyrer, 2023).

Trait psychologists prefer to use dimensions to replace all categories of PD (Krueger et al., 2018). They are not concerned about separating psychiatry from medicine – that may even be part of their agenda. Eventually they hope to conquer all of psychiatry for dimensional diagnosis, and might be expected to be sympathetic to systems that eschew categories. They consider those who want to retain categories to be "conservative." That is not a positive label in the academic world, where it tends to be attached to those who are skeptical of change.

As a lifelong gadfly, I am not used to be called conservative. But my colleagues and I, who work more with patients than with theories, find BPD to be a useful clinical construct. Thus, my view is that, at least for now, eliminating all PD categories would be a mistake. Most providers would need extra training to use the AMPD or the ICD-11. So at this point we need both categories and dimensions. I support the adoption of the AMPD as a clinically sensible compromise. No one has shown that a more radical change would help patients.

4.6 Borderline Personality Disorder: A Brief Summary

BPD is the most clinically important PD, but its label is a misnomer; there is no "border" on which to be borderline. (The historical explanation is that BPD was originally thought to be related to psychosis.) The diagnosis might better be described as *emotional dysregulation disorder*, since dysregulated emotions are its main feature. That might make BPD into a mood disorder, as once suggested by Tyrer (2014). But BPD has a number of features that go beyond mood instability and that fit better into the construct of personality disorder: widespread impulsivity, unstable relationships, and brief psychotic episodes that emerge under stress (Paris, 2020b). About half of these patients will hear critical voices when under stress, which is not true of any other PD.

BPD patients tend to present to emergency settings with suicidal ideas, self-harm (usually cutting), or with a suicide attempt (usually an overdose of pills). These symptoms are more common in women, but patients of both sexes can have problems with substance use. Emotional dysregulation feeds these fires and makes close relationships intense and unstable (Paris, 2020b, 2025).

What is most notable about BPD patients is how often they are acutely or chronically suicidal. That is the feature which attracted my interest as a young clinician. Most patients with BPD are young women, and the disorder becomes apparent in early adolescence (Kaess et al., 2014). Men with BPD can also be found in the community, but do not come as often for help (Trull et al., 2010). Men have more externalizing disorders such as substance use and antisocial behavior and are more often seen in clinics for those problems (Bozzatello et al., 2024).

These features do not make BPD patients popular with professionals who work in emergency settings. Since the ER is where people with BPD are at their worst, they may be viewed as "treatment resistant" or incurable. But that view has been revised on the basis of research. As Cohen pointed out long ago, clinicians have a bias to see more chronicity in their patients because they evaluate more of those who have not responded to treatment, as opposed to those who have remitted.

Long-term prospective studies have followed BPD patients for as long as 24 years, and most go into remission over time (Zanarini, 2018). And many stop meeting DSM criteria much sooner than that (Gunderson et al., 2011). Retrospective studies, such as the one carried out after 20 years by our research group, found a very similar pattern of recovery.

We now know that BPD begins early in adolescence (Kaess et al., 2014) and, in the vast majority of cases, the disorder remits by age 30–35 (Paris, 2020b). Some of these patients, even in the absence of treatment, recover as they mature. But we now have evidence-based and specialized psychotherapies that have been shown to be efficacious for this population (Paris, 2009a). This combination of dramatic symptoms but ultimate treatability has sparked interest among health care professionals in offering therapy for these patients. The severity of this disorder is why every conference on BPD treatment is fully subscribed by clinicians. But we can now be more optimistic about its prognosis.

Some years ago, I was part of a program sponsored by the National Institute of Mental Health (NIMH) designed to increase awareness of BPD by holding conferences in the USA, Canada, and the UK, in collaboration with family advocacy groups. Our message was that research shows that BPD patients are treatable and get better with time. I hope (but cannot prove) that education had some impact in reducing the stigma associated with BPD. This disorder is now more often recognized, and more patients are referred to specialized psychotherapy clinics.

In 2001, my team began by offering highly structured but brief treatment, mostly based on the principles of dialectical behavior therapy (DBT; Linehan, 1993). Our teams continue to offer treatment programs that combine group therapy (for teaching life skills) with individual therapy (for more personal problems). These programs offer several options for length of treatment, with the largest number treated for 12 weeks, and a smaller number for 6–12 months. Patients are asked to set goals as soon as they begin treatment. Therapy is partly based on psychoeducation – for emotion regulation, controlling impulsivity, and managing relationships. All patients are encouraged to prepare for discharge from the beginning of treatment, and to apply the skills they have learned on their own for at least six months after they leave the program.

Our program applies a model of *stepped care* (see Chapter 10), in which most patients are offered the 12-week program first, while those who did not benefit can return at a later point and be seen for 6–12 months (Paris, 2022a). We published results based on effectiveness data in a large sample of over 500 patients (Laporte et al., 2018) and are currently working to replicate and expand these findings. Combined with a satellite clinic at another hospital, we have been able to treat about 100 patients a year after a short wait. We do not claim to cure everyone, but that is not necessarily a goal either in psychiatry or in medicine. But at least two-thirds of our patients achieve a symptomatic remission. Crucially, treatment for BPD is now more accessible and has helped large numbers of patients to modify problematic traits and to overcome symptoms.

Not every treatment is simple or easy. BPD is associated with major "comorbidities," some of which are also diagnostic criteria for the PD. Substance use, if severe, can dominate a patient's life, and these patients may need to have their addiction treated first. Similarly, if there is access to a program for eating disorders, then severe anorexia nervosa and/or bulimia nervosa take priority. Some BPD patients (about a third) may also meet criteria for PTSD (Scheiderer et al., 2015). Nevertheless, as discussed in Chapters 1 and 2, exposure to trauma has a highly variable impact, and does not account for the wider range of psychopathology seen in BPD. That is why I do not refer BPD patients to "trauma-focused therapy," and why I am critical of the ICD-11 diagnosis of complex PTSD (Paris, 2023c).

As has often been reported, BPD has comorbidities with other PDs (Zanarini et al., 1998). An additional diagnosis of avoidant PD is a signal for treatment resistance, as it is associated with high social anxiety and isolation, leading to serious difficulty managing close relationships or a job. When present, these features make treatment more difficult

(Cramer et al., 2006). It is harder to get patients to take the risk of behavioral activation than to get them to stop behaviors that harm them.

The good news is that the majority of BPD patients get better with time. The other piece of good news is that they do well with a variety of therapies, most of which lead to similar outcomes. Meta-analyses confirm that specialized therapy is better than "treatment as usual" (Cristea et al., 2017).

The largest amount of research has been conducted on dialectical behavior therapy (DBT), and the results are generally good. But as shown by a Cochrane report (Storebø et al., 2018), the DBT method has not been found to be superior in head-to-head comparisons with other therapies.

The recently published revised Clinical Practice Guidelines (CPGs) for BPD from the American Psychiatric Association (Keepers et al., 2024) are a welcome development, and are a major improvement on a previous version dating from 2001. Along with roughly similar guidelines from the Cochrane Collaboration (Storebo et al., 2018), as well as from the National Institute for Clinical Excellence (2018), it is clear that psychotherapy is the treatment of choice, while pharmacological agents play only an adjunctive or minor role. Given these guidelines, I anticipate that a "borderline pattern" may still be recognized for some time to come.

I will not discuss the other PD categories in DSM-5-TR in any detail, as there is hardly any research on them. The AMPD has downplayed these diagnoses, and the ICD-11 drops them entirely. The exception is antisocial (or dissocial) PD. Clinicians will not see many patients with antisocial or psychopathic behaviors if they rarely seek treatment. While there has been less research on this clinical picture than on BPD, these patients, who are mostly male, are often found in the legal system or in addiction clinics (Black, 2024). There the focus is more likely on criminal behavior and/or substance use.

4.7 Personality, Health, and Success

In the heyday of psychoanalysis, it was common for patients to seek out therapy for life problems that may not be related to symptoms, but to marital conflicts, problems at work, or loneliness. My teachers thought that they could manage all these problems by reshaping a patient's personality. Needless to say, they had no proof for such a radical claim. Nonetheless, there is a good case for setting goals of less dramatic changes in personality. Using the FFM, it has been empirically shown that psychotherapy can, at least to some extent, modify trait profiles (Roberts et al., 2017). This usually involves reducing neuroticism while increasing agreeableness and conscientiousness.

These findings can be accounted for in part by current methods teaching patients to manage their emotions, or what has been called a "unified protocol" (UP; Barlow et al., 2020). This model is based on research showing that higher levels of neuroticism are associated with a wide range of mental disorders, marked by anxiety, depression, or dysregulated emotions. Reducing neuroticism is a central aim of most evidence-based psychotherapies.

By and large, it is better not to have high levels of neuroticism. It is also better to be mildly extraverted and reasonably agreeable, traits that support stable relationships. A higher level of conscientiousness is strongly associated with success in a career, and high levels also predict good health and longevity (Strickhouser et al., 2017).

To achieve personality change, therapists should not be overly ambitious. But what seem like small adjustments can go a long way. Misguided attempts to do too much for personality traits may explain why therapies go on for years (until funds run out). It also helps to explain why short-term therapies with a clear target are the only forms of psychological treatment that are evidence-based. Unfortunately, patients and therapists become accustomed to each other, even if the themes discussed in therapy keep repeating themselves. That is why the human bond that is the engine of change in therapy can eventually work against its own goals.

4.8 Mental Health Professionals and Personality Pathology

I have been told by clinical psychologists that I do much the same work as they do. But not all mental health professionals are interested in treating suicidal patients. Fortunately, I have led teams of psychologists, occupational therapists, and social workers who are comfortable with suicidality – as long as a psychiatrist has done a consultation or is on the treatment team. This experience has led to a somewhat different approach to suicide risk, as documented in my previous books (Paris, 2023b, 2024).

As a physician, I learned to accept that some patients will die in spite of treatment. Thus, I am somewhat less frightened of losing patients by suicide (see Chapter 8). Moreover, if patients do need medication (e.g., for insomnia), it is better for me to write the prescription than to farm it out to a physician who will overprescribe. I also have no problem with not prescribing or deprescribing, as I am aware of the limitations of current medications on the market. Moreover, there is little evidence that medications are needed for conditions that are commonly comorbid with BPD (Ribeiro et al., 2024). But there is a role for using antipsychotics in patients who have had brief psychotic episodes (Ingenhoven and Duivenvoorden, 2011).

One of the largest problems I see is the overuse of antidepressants in PD patients. I am almost never asked to consult on patients who are not already taking these agents. My experience with family doctors is that they routinely overprescribe because they follow algorithms for depression that recommend adding drugs with the aim of "augmentation." They are focusing on changes in mood or anxiety and missing the effects of personality.

Moreover, the reason I have always been against giving prescribing privileges to psychologists is *not* that they could not do just as well as physicians in conducting pharmacotherapy. Rather they would be likely to overprescribe, as I have often observed with nurse practitioners. But BPD patients don't benefit from antidepressants (Stoffers-Winterling et al., 2020), although by the time they see me, they may already have been tried on every drug on the market.

Patients with BPD should almost always be treated with evidence-based psychotherapy methods designed for this population (Storebo et al., 2018). Sadly, therapy of that kind is not readily available or well insured (see discussion in Chapter 7). Moreover, psychiatrists are also not always well trained to manage these cases. Another obstacle is that psychiatrists are often wary of patients with BPD, preferring to focus on what has been called "treatment resistant depression" (Gaynes et al., 2020). Some of my teachers who did offer psychotherapy found another way to avoid BPD – they did not reserve care for the most severe and complex patients, but took on less severely ill clients, and followed them for years.

I eventually concluded that psychiatry and clinical psychology are separate but overlapping domains, and that we should be working together in teams. I prefer to treat the most challenging patients, some of whom need management of medication, while others are encouraged to stop. As I became an experienced therapist, there was no reason to split the treatment.

Another obstacle for managing complex psychopathology is that treatment is often carried out in private offices. I have long thought that offices are not the best place to practice psychiatry (Paris et al., 2015b). Instead, we should be working with other mental health professionals in hospitals or clinics with group practices (see Chapter 9 for further discussion). It is hard to manage unusually difficult patients without a team behind you (Linehan, 1993).

My career has been located almost entirely in public sector hospitals, as well as in a mental health clinic for university students. In these settings, I worked with clinical psychologists with whom I would meet for weekly team meetings. This model was, at least for me, the best of all possible worlds.

These reflections lead me to thoughts about the future of psychiatry. Our hard-earned skills should not be limited to consultations followed by 15-minute checkups. We are trained to carry out psychotherapy and can expand those skills by practicing them with PD patients, and/or supporting other professionals who have a similar interest in this population.

More generally, psychiatrists should not be treating patients with mild problems. There is a veritable army of therapists in the community ready to take those tasks on. The main obstacle is that these services may not be insured, making access difficult. There is a great demand for psychotherapy that is not being met by our current health system. This situation is one of many casualties of the stigma of mental illness. It is not the only one (failure to provide adequate support to psychotic patients is another). But it is still a tragedy and a lost opportunity for societies that value mental and physical health.

Answer to Unanswered Question #4
Behind the symptoms that are used to define mental disorders are personality traits that are measures of vulnerability. When amplified, they can lead to personality disorders. We now have effective methods of treating these disorders, particularly BPD. But doing so requires psychiatrists to conduct or to refer for psychotherapy, preferably in multidisciplinary teams.

Evidence-Based Psychiatry

Unanswered Question #5: Is it possible to ensure a broad commitment among clinicians to evidence-based practice?

5.1 The Rise of Evidence-Based Mental Health Practice

When I was a student, we were expected to adopt the opinions of our senior professors. They were never asked to present any evidence in support of their views. After all, gray hairs must be a sign of extensive clinical experience. Moreover, if you openly disagreed, there could be consequences. Teachers saw me as a rebel for being a gadfly (which I still am).

I spent a year as a resident on an in-patient ward where patients with severe mental disorders were kept in hospital for months to allow for intensive psychotherapy. I thought these patients were being made worse by regressive hospitalizations that put the rest of their life on hold, and said so. But these differences were not settled by asking what research shows. (There wasn't any data on this issue at the time.) Medicine had a military style of practice, and asking for empirical evidence about treatment was seen as a sign of disloyalty. Today, the expense of admission, and the backlog of patients held over in emergency rooms waiting for a bed, means that only the most acutely ill patients stay in hospital, and are discharged earlier.

Moreover, health care has adopted a very different philosophy. Medicine, psychiatry, and clinical psychology are more based on research. But not everything that clinicians do can be tested for effectiveness. There are many times when evidence for or against an intervention is entirely lacking. Nonetheless, clinicians should remain committed to science.

A movement for *Evidence-Based Medicine* (EBM; Sackett et al., 1996), founded in Oxford, UK, and Hamilton, Canada, has had the support of most academics. Its premise is straightforward – medical treatments should be supported by the best available evidence. But we should not change our practice based on the results of single studies, which may not be replicated (Ioannidis, 2005, 2012). Researchers carry out meta-analyses because the weight of data from multiple sources is much more valid, and more convincing.

Evidence-based psychiatry (Gray, 2008) is the application of EBM to the specialty. Its recommendations can be accessed by mental health clinicians in several ways. In the UK, a quarterly journal, *Evidence-Based Mental Health*, now renamed *BMJ Mental Health*, is sponsored by the British Journal of Psychiatry, the Royal College of Psychiatrists, and the British Psychological Association. It is devoted to reviewing and integrating data about the efficacy of treatments in clinical trials, and their effectiveness in real-world clinical settings.

Another major source for decisions about the treatment is the Cochrane Collaboration reports that are regularly published and available on the web. Cochrane is the most conservative source, which is what I like about it. Actually, almost half of systematic reviews related to clinical practice in medicine fail to confirm that treatments are effective (Villas Boas et al., 2013). But while some may worry about "therapeutic nihilism," I am more concerned about prescribing treatments that don't work.

Then there are Clinical Practice Guidelines (CPGs), published by professional associations in different countries. In the US, CPGs are sponsored by the American Psychiatric Association, and a list of Empirically Supported Therapies (ESTs) is offered by the American Psychological Association. In the UK, treatment guidelines are the responsibility of the National Institute for Clinical Excellence (NICE). Several other countries, including Canada, publish their own CPGs. Finally, clinicians can read journals that publish systematic reviews and meta-analyses. I find *World Psychiatry*, freely available online, to be particularly helpful, since it publishes many systematic reviews and meta-analyses, on which clinicians should rely.

Let us consider once more the problem of a replication crisis in both medical and psychological research (Ritchie, 2020). One should never trust the findings of a single study, as there are so many ways that they may not (or never) be replicated. The problems range from poor methods to doubtful interpretations of data. Among the most common problems is "p-hacking," in which only statistically significant findings ($p < .05$) are reported. Even the most prestigious journals have been seriously embarrassed after publishing articles that were seriously flawed. Again, my advice is to always wait for replications, meta-analyses, or systematic reviews. Moreover, keep in mind that a relationship between two variables can meet the target of $p < .05$ but still not apply to most members of the population under study.

Most psychiatrists and clinical psychologists subscribe, at least in principle, to evidence-based practice. One exception is a Canadian colleague (Gupta, 2014), who published a book-length critique of EBM in psychiatry. Her argument was that if too little is known about mental illness, giving priority to RCTs and meta-analyses limits research by asking the wrong questions, making EBM less than ethical as a basis for patient care. I strongly disagree, because I have seen the alternative – every man (or woman) for themselves. I also disagree with Gupta that qualitative research can be used to ask different but more pertinent research questions. At best, that method can suggest hypotheses that can then be tested quantitatively. I have reviewed qualitative studies for journals, and view many of them as little but collections of anecdotes drawn from small samples. If you fail to quantify what you observe, you are not doing good science.

In principle then, evidence-based psychiatry should dominate treatment choices for all of us. The question is how many practicing mental health clinicians actually make use of evidence in their practice. Although availability of research on the internet is a boon, if you don't work in academia, you have to pay for access to journals. Moreover, no one funds the time needed to find, read, and process these recommendations. Instead, many clinicians depend on packaged advice in Continuing Medical Education (CME, mostly consisting of conferences), as required by licensing bodies, but often sponsored by the pharmaceutical industry. In the case of psychiatrists, as long as Pharma pays the bill, many CME events suffer from serious conflicts of interest.

Like many others, I found it was possible to attend the annual meeting of the American Psychiatric Association without paying for a single meal, and to collect pens marked with the name of a drug. This situation is now better, but possibly only because there are fewer new agents on the market. Psychologists don't have to worry about the pharmaceutical industry, but what they hear about psychotherapy mostly comes from experts who want to promote books.

5.2 To What Extent Are Clinicians Committed to Evidence-Based Practice?

Some of my colleagues consider CPGs to be a source of wisdom. But these reports are written by committees of experts who may have their own axe to grind, even if they need to reach a consensus with other members. These biases and ideological commitments tend to make experts overly optimistic. That is why some researchers have proposed tools to make CPGs more trustworthy (Brouwers et al., 2020; Guerra-Farfan et al., 2023).

And that is why I have long admired the caution of reports from the Cochrane Collaboration. Some find these reports overly cautious. But as I am more worried about unsupported enthusiasm, I want the bar to be high.

Research to determine whether or not practitioners carry out evidence-based practice in the prescription of medications or psychotherapies to treat mental disorders is rare. We know from a large survey that psychiatrists in the US do not follow the algorithms of the DSM manual when making a diagnosis (First et al., 2014). I doubt that the situation is better when clinicians choose treatment options. Moreover, physicians who are insufficiently skeptical of the industry are more likely to prescribe new medications that are no better than older ones, just more expensive (Wazana, 2000).

By and large, only academics follow the research literature closely. Even then, they mostly read articles in their own narrow domain. We do not have good data on how much clinicians in practice know, and how much they apply their reading or what they learn from attending conferences. What they hear may or may not be valid or reliable. Even if it is, we do not know whether the advice they get from attending conferences is applied to their practice – or even remembered a few weeks later (Cervero and Gaines, 2015).

When CME for psychiatrists is paid for by Pharma, and when the experts who speak receive money for doing so, it might be better to avoid these meetings entirely. In psychopharmacology, a skeptical attitude about the claims of new drugs on the market should always be warranted. My view is that we should prescribe older drugs that are just as effective but much cheaper for patients. In psychotherapy, the largest problem is the translation from research to practice. There is little evidence that therapists pay serious attention to what science is trying to tell them.

Twenty years ago, Norcross et al. (2007) raised nine questions about how much evidence-based practice affects the provision of psychotherapies (that also apply to pharmacotherapy).

The first is what qualifies as evidence of effective practice – research findings or patient preferences? Many patients come these days asking for a specific treatment, which may or may not be the best choice. I would say that we have a responsibility to inform our patients about what research does or does not support.

The second is what kind of research is strong enough to be put into practice – is it randomized clinical trials, effectiveness studies without randomization, or some other measure? I would vote for a confluence of evidence that all points in the same direction.

A third issue is whether manualization of treatment improves outcome – most research says it does not (Truijens et al., 2019). Chapter 7 will review data showing good reason to conclude that the personal skills of therapists are more crucial than their theories or specific methods.

The fourth is that while RCTs have many advantages, they are not always generalizable. That is because they are carried out on selected samples that are not representative of the patients whom clinicians see in practice (Hollon and Wampold, 2009). Our treatments need to be shown to work in a real-world setting by effectiveness studies, but they are much less common.

The fifth is how change and outcome should be measured – symptom relief, patient satisfaction, or evidence of better functioning. Since results may differ in each domain, all should be assessed.

The sixth concerns the effects of theoretical allegiances. Most research fails to find differences in outcome when comparing therapies based on different theories (Wampold and Imel, 2015).

The seventh is whether empirically supported treatments actually have a better outcome. This has not been shown by research (Westen and Bradley, 2005). Again, theory and methods are less important than skills. A similar conclusion arises from what psychotherapy research tells us about efficacy, that is, that there are few differences in efficacy between competing methods. But we need not downplay the requirement for evidence: The importance of common factors need not stand in the way of research on more specific methods.

The eighth is whether current methods are suitable for minority populations. In an era where delivering care to minorities is a priority, this subject requires more research.

The ninth is how easily efficacious therapies can be translated into normal practice. In Chapter 7, I will discuss how well-researched treatments can be brief, and are less than useful if they go on too long and are too expensive.

We are not yet doing a good enough job at ensuring that treatments, whether biological or psychological, are evidence-based. We should not endorse prescribing the latest drugs on the market without data on efficacy and side effects, or the free-for-all in which hundreds of psychotherapies compete for the spotlight. Some clinicians just want "to do their own thing," and they may claim that research data supports their choices. But we have twenty-odd antidepressants to choose from, all of which only help a little more than half the patients for whom they are prescribed (see Chapter 6).

The problem is that mental health clinicians are not being held accountable for their choices, especially in private practice. Academics are more likely to be evidence-based, to work in multidisciplinary teams, and to discuss new developments with colleagues. Those who work alone in an office are more at risk of offering options that are well marketed but add little to their toolbox. These range from polypharmacy prescriptions that are renewed for years, to psychotherapies that invite patients to spend years blaming their parents for traumatizing them.

Given opportunities to follow the evidence, why do so many mental health clinicians decline to offer what science tells them is safest and best? Lilienfeld et al. (2013) identified obstacles underpinning resistance to the evidence-based practice of psychotherapy; these include (a) naïve realism, in which clinicians conclude erroneously that change is due to their interventions rather than to other explanations; (b) misconceptions regarding the causal primacy of early experiences; (c) statistical misunderstandings regarding the application of findings in groups to individuals; (d) placing the burden of proof on skeptics rather than on proponents of therapies; and (e) discomfort with an increasingly technical outcome literature.

Behind these factors is the tendency of all kinds of mental health clinicians to have an ideological and/or a sentimental loyalty to their teachers. Moreover, in a competitive market, practitioners tend to define themselves in a way that meets the expectations of their society. In pharmacology, patients expect a prescription and may demand one. In psychotherapy, some modern therapists have been rebranding themselves as trauma-informed specialists. With all these forces in play, following research guidelines may not be a priority.

These problems ultimately derive from the culture of mental health care. They begin early on, when clinicians are trained by teachers with strong theoretical beliefs that prevent them from embracing evidence-based practice. What academics should be teaching is that it is best to be skeptical about the efficacy of any drug or any psychotherapy, especially when they are new.

Ioannidis (2017) has examined the question of whether EBM has been hijacked by industry for profit, and concludes (p. 11):

> [A] number of criticisms that have been raised against evidence-based medicine, such as focusing on benefits and ignoring adverse events; being interested in averages and ignoring the wide variability in individual risks and responsiveness; ignoring clinician-patient interaction and clinical judgement; leading to some sort of reductionism; and falling prey to corruption from conflicts of interest.... [N]one of these deficiencies are necessarily inherent to evidence-based medicine. In fact, work in evidence-based medicine has contributed a lot towards minimizing these deficiencies in medical research and medical care.

5.3 A Golden Age for Evidence-Based Practice?

In spite of all the problems this chapter has raised, we are living in a new era, a potentially golden age for evidence-based psychiatry and empirically supported psychotherapies. I say this because I was trained in a different time and only adopted the EBM model in middle age. In the past, medications and therapies were often chosen through hallway discussions, which have their place, but are no substitute for consulting the research literature.

When I look back on how gullible I was in the past, I wonder what I could have been thinking (or not thinking). Some people feel apologetic when they compare psychiatry to other branches of medicine, in which research has uncovered the causes of many diseases, more often leading to specific treatment choices. But I prefer to compare psychiatry with other disciplines, such as the social sciences, that lie on the boundaries between empiricism and theory. I see these domains as lacking a strong commitment to scientific rigor.

My teachers had impressive certainty, combined with powerful rhetoric. If you disagreed with them, they would say, "That is my clinical experience." But they had little else to back up their ideas. I am reminded of the current trend to give some priority to what patients think, that is, "lived experience" (Yeo et al., 2022). It is useful to consider patients as partners in evaluating treatment, but their ideas about what ails them and what they need may only be anecdotes. Treatment can be consistent with patient values but still be evidence-based.

Nobody today would believe some of the fantastic ideas I heard from my teachers, such as that psychoses are the result of bad parenting (Dolnick, 1998). It took decades to prove these ideas wrong (and harmful), but they are no longer popular – except in the cultish fringes of psychiatry.

No doubt some of our current beliefs will eventually be found to be equally absurd. And the practice of blaming families for mental illness is far from over. Today our trainees are encouraged to read the research literature before coming to premature conclusions. In particular, firm conclusions cannot be derived from single studies. For this reason, I advise students to respect the findings of meta-analyses. I am fortunate to have had a career in an academic setting, where science can, at least in principle, trump opinion. But these new ways of thinking are trickling down to the world of office practice, where beliefs without evidence have so often ruled.

5.4 Integrating EBM Principles into the Practice of Psychiatry

Practitioners need not be working alone. If they treat patients in offices outside hospitals, it would be better for them to join a group practice with other colleagues. They need to avoid being isolated in their offices. Then they would have easy access to second opinions on difficult cases. Moreover, this structure is highly suitable for learning about research findings, without the various conflicts of interest that have undermined current methods of continuing medical education. Working in an academic setting, I have greatly benefited from attending journal clubs with colleagues and students, as well as study groups examining how research can be applied to clinical problems. I would not have been able to write books such as this one if I did not have collegial support, learning how to search the literature and to apply it to treating patients. Even if not all my colleagues are equally curious, this is a wise investment of time that can enrich clinical work and reduce the loneliness of solo practice. Given the emotional demands on us, our work can be stressful and carry a real risk of "burnout" (Bykov et al., 2022).

5.5 The Broader Range of Evidence-Based Principles

When I once explained to a friend that medicine is more based in science, he asked, "Do you mean to say it has not been relying on evidence all along?" Unfortunately, that is indeed the case. And psychiatry is neither better nor worse than other specialties.

When I look back on my medical-school training, students were not taught to become critical readers of the scientific literature. In fact, during four years as a medical student, I was *never* directed by any teacher to read scientific articles. Perhaps, given the low standards of much that was being published in those days, students may not have missed out. Some years ago, I went to the library to see what leading psychiatric journals in the middle of the 20th century were publishing. Most of these articles reported either clinical impressions or case series to support pet theories. Almost all were innocent of statistics.

Residency training was not much better for my generation to learn how to think scientifically. There were no journal clubs in those days, and residents were not taught how to interpret quantitative research studies. A few years into my career, I was asked to direct the training of residents at a university teaching hospital. The first thing I did was to start a journal club. Half a century later, that format remains a valued and popular part of psychiatric education.

Even today, I find a certain level of resistance to evidence-based psychiatry. It comes from a small number of clinicians still on faculty who were trained in specific methods. But another source of opposition comes from the idea that the "lived experience" of our patients is just as important as data. I oppose this trend, which is little but a return to a time when opinion was more important than measurement.

The principles of relying on an evidence base are also important for academic disciplines in the social sciences that lie outside of medicine. One of these is psychology, which should be a basic science for psychiatry. However, psychology is a very broad field, and there is a large gap between how clinicians and researchers come to conclusions. Another domain that can be quantitative is sociology, which has a tradition of large-scale surveys. (Economics and political science also use survey data but are not relevant to psychiatry.) The outlier is cultural anthropology, whose tradition of "participant obser-vation" fails to turn reports of interviews into reliable data. Like "lived experience" in mental health, it leads to doubtful conclusions about society and culture.

These comparisons with other disciplines make me conclude that psychiatry is at least as evidence-based as other domains that study the complexities of human behavior. If we have not reached the same level of evidence-based practice as has general medicine, that is the most likely reason.

Answer to Unanswered Question #5
Psychiatrists, clinical psychologists, and other mental health professionals can offer evidence-based treatment, but our clinical culture needs to change. The model of a solo practitioner working in an office with little input from what research is telling practitioners is outdated and problematic.

Psychopharmacology

Unanswered Question #6: Why is treatment with psychopharmacology, after dramatic advances 50 years ago, in a state of suspended animation?

A "psychopharmacological revolution" occurred between the 1950s and 1970s. Healey (2004) described it as one of the greatest triumphs in the history of psychiatry and medicine. As a medical student and a resident, I lived through this era and found it inspiring.

New medications were introduced that controlled psychotic episodes, that prevented hospitalizations, and that allowed patients to be discharged much earlier. These agents, originally developed in France, became standard around the globe within a few years (Lehmann, 1958). As a result, mental hospitals emptied out, and many were eventually demolished.

Yet that was only a partial victory, and its promises of comprehensive community-based care were never realized. Not all patients, especially those diagnosed with schizo-phrenia, did well living in the community, and those who did not take their medications regularly often relapsed (Angst, 1988). Later, long-acting antipsychotics were introduced that could be given by regular injections. But patients still have to show up for that choice to be effective.

I volunteered at a mental hospital for several years as a medical student. A group of us founded an "Arts and Sciences Club" for convalescing patients. When I was a resident in psychiatry, I spent a year at this hospital, where long admissions made it into a kind of community. But now that we had access to drugs that could control psychosis, the mental hospital was never the same.

A second breakthrough occurred a few years later, when lithium began to be used for manic episodes. This was a slow process. Lithium treatment was discovered in Australia (Cade, 1949), studied in Denmark (Schou et al., 1954), and tested in Canada (Kingstone, 1960). Why was this powerful agent slow to catch on? Perhaps pharmaceutical com-panies were reluctant to market a simple salt. In 1969, as a resident, I was one of the early physicians at a general hospital to prescribe lithium, and to observe its almost miraculous ability to control manic episodes and prevent relapses in bipolar patients. This success was so complete that the first patient to whom I gave lithium, after 25 previous admissions, responded in a few days and was never hospitalized again.

The third breakthrough was the development of tricyclic antidepressants (Healey, 2004). These drugs (now replaced by specific serotonin reuptake inhibitors or SSRIs) are often effective against depression. They are not as miraculous as lithium, and have a strong placebo response, only yielding remission in a little more than half of cases (Del Re et al., 2013). Today, these drugs are being prescribed routinely, but are most useful for a subgroup with severe depression (Fournier et al., 2010).

In the 1970s, just as neuroscience was rapidly expanding, the psychopharmacological revolution ran out of steam. Today's antipsychotics and antidepressants have different side effects but are no more effective than older medications. (The one drug that has made the most difference for managing psychosis is clozapine, to be discussed in Section 6.2.)

The pharmaceutical industry keeps trying to convince us otherwise. Many psychiatrists prescribe the latest "copycat" medications in the hope that they will be more effective, or just to try them out. These agents have similar mechanisms of action and only minor differences in chemical structure. Actually, the one thing you can be sure of newer agents is that they will be more expensive. It is a matter of record that shortly after older drugs go out of patent, even without any change in efficacy, their sales rapidly plummet (Feldman and Frondorf, 2017).

The pharmaceutical industry is not a charitable foundation, but a business built on profit. That is why physicians see fewer of their representatives knocking on our doors. A lack of progress in developing new drugs for psychiatry eventually led industry to focus on other problems.

6.1 The Corruption of Psychiatry by Industry

As a witness to the psychopharmacological revolution, I was sympathetic to the idea that physicians and industry should be partners in treating the mentally ill. However, slowly but surely, I was forced to change my mind. The pioneering days were over. And since mental disorders of one kind or other affect so many people, the profits to be made by pharma have been enormous.

The result has been the corruption of psychiatry. Many experts took large sums of money from industry to promote the latest agents, even when they were no better than older ones. Attendees at conferences were impressed by beautifully crafted colored slides claiming to show how drugs stabilize brain synapses. Moreover, over-medication became common, reflecting a shift in psychiatry to a model based on what was believed to be neuroscience. I once asked a psychiatry professor at a leading university what he does when antidepressants fail to help patients. His answer was that he would consult a colleague specializing in psychopharmacology. But doing so would almost be a guarantee of polypharmacy. When I have needed a consultation on my own patients, I have preferred asking colleagues who have expertise in a wide variety of treatments.

In recent decades, we have learned of scandals in which well-known psychiatrists earned millions of dollars for serving as "key opinion leaders" for the pharmaceutical industry. As one recent survey confirms, these payments are not given to ordinary clinicians but to academic leaders (Havlik et al., 2025). These experts are often the star attractions of conferences to promote continuing medical education (CME), where they promote the latest drugs. That is what they are paid for.

In past years, you could not go to the annual meeting of the American Psychiatric Association (APA) without picking up many goodies paid for by the industry. Few of us were able to resist these "gifts," ranging from pens to dinners at expensive restaurants.

Some of my colleagues even accepted free travel to attend these meetings. (When the conference was held in New York, some psychiatrists were given tickets to Broadway shows.)

One of my colleagues posed the question in a frequently cited article: "When is a gift just a gift?." The answer is that all gifts from the industry have strings attached. Research shows that even without a quid pro quo, accepting gifts, even small ones, has a direct effect on the prescription practice of those who accept them. These norms also affect training in psychiatry, where pizza may be provided for residents attending Journal Clubs. While on a visit to another university in Canada, I attended a trainee "awards night" and was shocked when certificates were given out – not by faculty, but by pharmaceutical representatives.

I can report that this situation has now improved, at least where I work. One reason may be that there have been few truly new drugs in recent years. We therefore have less contact with industry than in the past. If psychiatrists go to a dinner meeting, they pay out of pocket (or, if they work in a hospital, draw on funds pooled from clinical income). Today, for academics, every presentation at a conference, publication, or work on a committee requires filling out a detailed statement on potential conflicts of interest. (These forms require us to state whether we could have a conflict if we receive royalties for writing books for mental health clinicians – including this one.) These stricter rules may reduce the frequency of corruption among the well-known psychiatrists who became millionaires through payments from industry.

Drugs are not cheap. The pharmaceutical industry claims that this is because they invest heavily in research. But they spend much more on marketing. Industry also claims that they are producing better drugs than ever, but that is false. We could do about as well if the medications of 50 years ago were all we had. The main difference is that serious side effects are less common, which is why specific serotonin uptake inhibitors (SSRIs) are favored by primary care providers (Arroll et al., 2016).

6.2 Pharmacological Treatment of Psychoses

Psychiatrists often treat mental illness successfully – in spite of not knowing the mechanism behind their tools. Of course, that is much better than not having anything useful to offer.

Psychoses such as schizophrenia have been a mainly positive story. Psychotic episodes can usually be controlled, and we now use "second generation" drugs with fewer neurological side effects. Unfortunately, these agents do not target all the symptoms of schizophrenia. Moreover, newer drugs can lead to a "metabolic syndrome" that resembles diabetes (Carli et al., 2021).

Patients who do not respond to standard antipsychotic medications may do better if prescribed clozapine. This is an old drug that was revived, and it can work when other agents fail (Fakra and Azorin, 2012; Rubio and Kane, 2020; Warnez and Alessi-Severini, 2014). Clozapine was once touted by *Time* magazine as a new day for the treatment of schizophrenia. There is also evidence that patients are less likely to die by suicide if they take clozapine (Meltzer et al., 2003). Managing this drug and its side effects (e.g., white blood cell reduction) does, however, require close monitoring.

Our ability to manage bipolar disorder is a parallel story – one of partial but significant success. We do not yet understand why a simple molecule can yield such amazing results. Antipsychotics also control manic symptoms, but patients tend to relapse and can have further episodes even when taking them.

Lithium always was, and still is, the best choice for mania, mainly because relapses are fewer (Geddes et al., 2004; Rybakowski, 2020). Due to the side effects of lithium, patients today may be prescribed anticonvulsant mood stabilizers instead – such as valproate and lamotrigine, but that choice risks more relapses. Also, lithium lowers the high rate of suicide in bipolar patients, and nothing else does (Cipriani et al., 2013). The introduction of lithium was a landmark in modern psychopharmacology, but this agent needs to be prescribed more often (Rybakowski, 2020). But it has to be closely monitored to manage its side effects.

6.3 Antidepressants

The efficacy of antidepressants is more mixed. Results vary from dramatic to none at all, and agents often lack large advantages over placebos (Kirsch, 2009). Their margin of efficacy decreases over time, particularly once drugs are no longer new on the market (Khan and Brown, 2015). This does not mean that antidepressants are ineffective, but that they are not consistently effective.

Today, antidepressants are being prescribed much more often, and are now being taken by about 15% of the population in the USA (National Center for Health Statistics, 2020). Prescription levels in the UK and Canada are similar. Physicians today prescribe SSRIs instead of tricyclics (older drugs that can be fatal if patients overdose on as little as one week's supply).

Antidepressants are a key tool for psychiatry, but do not necessarily yield a full remission of depressive symptoms (Mojtabai et al., 2021; Rush, 2023). We do not know why these drugs are effective, or why they can be ineffective. The idea that serotonin levels account for depression has not been proven, and there is even some evidence for the efficacy of drugs that do not affect serotonin (Moncrieff et al., 2023). Given strong placebo effects, one can be fooled by early responses that are not stable over time.

Another reason for inconsistent results in treatment is that major depression is being overdiagnosed (see Chapter 2). Thus, among the deeper reasons for a lack of progress is that we do not know how these drugs work in the brain, and that we lack a useful typology of depression.

Systematic reviews of efficacy of medications for depression have not yielded strong support for their routine use (Heingartner and Plöderl, 2022). One very large meta-analysis reported that at least half of patients improve with these prescriptions, with an odds ratio of about 2.0 above and beyond placebo (Cipriani et al., 2018). However, it is difficult to identify responders in advance. Data from effectiveness trials in the real world of clinical practice can help. The Sequenced Treatment Alternatives to Relieve Depression (STAR*D; Rush, 2023) found that randomized clinical trials of efficacy had overestimated their potency in practice, and that treatment resistance is common. These effectiveness studies have examined that real-world outcomes in depression are more representative of clinical reality than clinical trials that only include patients who volunteer to be randomized.

These problems have led to a search for alternative methods of treatment (Njenga et al., 2024). Only about half of depressed patients achieve remission with drug treatment alone. While a remission rate of 50% could be satisfactory in some domains of medicine, we need more consistent results. We are still left with a large population of depressed patients requiring different treatments.

Given such an uncertain response, why is such a large percentage of the population taking SSRIs? A good number of patients do respond to them. But well-supported alternatives are expensive and not widely available. As Chapter 7 will show, access to psychotherapy is problematic. A prescription costs a lot less. Moreover, once patients start taking antidepressants, they are afraid to stop them. The physicians who provide these medications are also afraid to deprescribe them.

Today the main alternatives in the face of treatment-resistant depression involve pharmacological programs based on switching or augmenting. The most usual alternative is to switch to another antidepressant, even though there is only weak empirical support for doing so. Research has failed to show that any one SSRI is better than any other (Cipriani et al., 2018), and that outcomes are much the same (Del Re et al., 2013). It may be worth trying to switch once, but not several times. Switching is also open to placebo effects that may not last. There is also no good evidence that so-called dual mechanism agents (that affect both serotonin and norepinephrine) such as venlafaxine are any more effective than SSRIs (Connolly and Thase, 2011).

The other option is *augmentation*. Prescribers may choose a low-dose antipsychotic with fewer side effects. However, the most popular choices are problematic. Aripiprazole has extrapyramidal side effects, while quetiapine, even in a low dose, can lead to a "metabolic syndrome" (Newcomer and Haupt, 2006). While some patients benefit from these combinations, outcomes are far from consistent (Connolly and Thase, 2011). Another more recent drug is ketamine, given by infusion (Smith-Apeldoorn et al., 2022). However, that treatment is still at an experimental stage, and its effects may only be temporary (Dean et al., 2021).

This failure to respond to multiple trials of antidepressants has been called *treatment resistance* (Gaynes et al., 2020). But we should be asking what we mean by "treatment." There are also non-pharmacological options. Some involve electrical stimulation of the brain. In melancholic depression, electroconvulsive therapy (ECT) can yield rapid results (UK ECT Review Group, 2003). We do not know why it works, but ECT might be compared with a restart on a computer. ECT is probably the most effective treatment in all of psychiatry. Unfortunately, due to stigma, a history of past overuse, hostility in the media, and lack of a theory, ECT is underutilized in psychiatry (Paris, 2022d). It should be the first choice for treatment-resistant depression (Trifu et al., 2021).

Another option is Transcranial Magnetic Stimulation (TMS), in which seizures are not required, but in which specific areas are targeted by electrodes on the scalp (Brini et al., 2023; Hyde et al., 2022). Although TMS has been supported by some research (Perera et al., 2016), it is expensive and not widely available.

Psychotherapy is not routinely offered to depressed patients. As Chapter 7 will show, many of these methods have strong evidence for efficacy. But its cost and a spotty insurance system are major factors working against wider application.

Finally, it is noteworthy that many depressions resolve naturalistically after a few months. It is therefore hard to know whether a recent change to a different antidepressant is more effective, whether psychotherapy is working, or whether what we are seeing is a gradual but naturalistic recovery. By the time it takes to try all the alternatives, you can't really know if treatments have done the work.

6.4 Brief Comments on Other Methods of Psychopharmacology

Benzodiazepines were introduced over 60 years ago and are currently used by about 5% of the population (Olfson et al., 2015). There is a danger of addiction in some patients – these agents are cross-tolerant with alcohol and can lead to habituation with continuous use. For treatment of chronic insomnia, there are better choices (De Crescenzo et al., 2022), such as zopiclone or sedating antidepressants. There is also good evidence for psychotherapy in insomnia, and options based on cognitive therapy are now freely available online (Cunningham and Shapiro, 2018).

Stimulants, mostly derived from amphetamines, are widely offered these days for patients with a diagnosis of ADHD, and their use has greatly increased (Olfson et al., 2013). As discussed in Chapter 2, there are good reasons to be cautious about making an ADHD diagnosis. We also do not know how serious could be cardiovascular effects after taking stimulants for years or decades (Zhang et al., 2024).

"Mood stabilizers" were originally developed as anticonvulsants, but this class of drugs is wrongly named. They should be reserved for bipolar patients (type I or type II) who do not tolerate lithium (Kishi et al., 2021). These agents may be used to treat mood swings of all kinds, but are not effective for personality disorders. Keep in mind that brief mood swings, lasting hours or at most a day, are common features of PDs that can be managed in psychotherapy (Linehan, 1993). Mistaken diagnoses can lead to mistaken treatments.

Some other developments are worthy of note. Addiction psychiatrists are prescribing naltrexone, best known as the antidote to an overdose of opiates. Along with similar agents, this agent can reduce craving for drugs (O'Malley et al., 2002).

Psychedelics are still an experimental therapy. These agents have not been approved for PTSD in the USA, but reviews thus far state that there is too little data to reach a conclusion (Muttoni et al., 2019; Yaden et al., 2024). It is too soon to tell if these agents are useful for mental disorders.

6.5 Why Psychiatrists Prescribe Too Many Drugs

For many years, anti-psychiatry activists picketed every annual meeting of the APA, accusing us of "drugging" patients. (They were sponsored by the Scientology cult.) I am a critic of overreliance on psychopharmacology but am also a strong supporter of medication where the evidence supports it.

There is little doubt that psychiatry has a major problem with overprescription, as well as multiple prescriptions. These practices lead to *polypharmacy*, with doubtful efficacy and the certainty of a heavy load of side effects. As the saying goes, "if all you have is a hammer, everything looks like a nail." Psychiatrists whose main skill is a prescription may be following this rule. If you are uninterested in psychotherapy, and/ or have little recent experience with it, you will pull out your prescription pad with every patient you see. That practice is further reinforced by the perception of many psychiatrists that their identity as a professional is bound up with neuroscience.

So what happens when medication is not effective? In principle, this scenario should launch a rethink about diagnosis and treatment. Yet switching and augmentation, each of which postpones reevaluation of the diagnosis, can go on for some time. I cannot tell how often I have heard patients with PDs describe this sequence, sometimes running through almost every agent on the market. It is not widely recognized that patients with comorbid PDs do not respond well to antidepressants (Mercer et al., 2009; Van and Kool, 2018). That may at least partially explain why treatment resistance is so common. At the same time, PDs often go underdiagnosed and undertreated.

Once again, too many psychiatrists have bought in to the mantra that all mental disorders are brain disorders. Yet that point of view is largely correct for schizophrenia and bipolar disorder. (Failure to medicate these patients is now an invitation to a lawsuit.) But it is not correct for depression. This heterogenous disorder, in spite of being ubiquitous in practice, does not respond consistently to any single method of treatment. Depression usually requires more than a prescription. As Chapter 7 will show, a large proportion of these patients benefit from a different prescription – for psychotherapy.

Answer to Unanswered Question #6
Psychiatry made great progress in pharmacotherapy 50 years ago, but there have been no major breakthroughs since. Nor is there currently a good reason to expect that newer drugs could lead to a second psychopharmacological revolution any time soon.

Psychotherapy

Unanswered Question #7: What is the role of psychotherapy in psychiatric practice, and should medical practitioners still be offering it?

7.1 The Decline of Psychotherapy in Psychiatry

In the mind of the public, psychiatrists may still be seen as mind doctors – physicians whose main skill lies in psychotherapy. But in the last few decades, they have largely stopped offering this kind of treatment (Olfson et al., 2024). Psychotherapy is now more likely to be provided by other mental health professionals (Olfson et al., 2025), while the modern practice of psychiatry is dominated by prescriptions. What used to be a 50-minute hour of listening and commenting has now often been reduced to a 15-minute checkup for medication.

But evidence-based psychotherapy has an enormous body of research supporting it (Markham et al., 2021). Psychological therapies have also been shown to be at least as effective as drug treatment for anxiety and depression (Cuijpers et al., 2025), and has a unique role in managing other disorders, including substance use (Galanter and Kleber, 2011), eating disorders (Monteleone and Abbate-Daga, 2024), and personality disorders (Paris, 2025). These conclusions, however, only apply to evidence-based therapies; many methods on the market have never been subject to clinical trials and are only backed up by books written by their developers. We should no more prescribe untested therapies than untested drugs.

But why did our specialty retreat from spending more time talking to patients? There are two main reasons. First, the way psychiatry is practiced reflects the rise of neuroscience as its dominant paradigm. Many psychiatrists today consider themselves not experts on the workings of the mind, but on psychopharmacology. And their practice has become more similar to what internists do. This part of the explanation for the decline of psychotherapy in psychiatry concerns the identity of our profession. Psychiatrists seek the same level of respect accorded to other medical specialists. They do not want to be seen as clinical psychologists who just happen to have been medically trained. By defining their practice as an application of neuroscience, they hope to find a unique niche.

The second part of the explanation has to do with economics. If you see four patients in an hour, you make much more money than if you only see one. Moreover, few patients can afford to pay large sums every month out of pocket. Sadly, insurance for psychotherapy is spotty in most countries. Where I work, psychiatrists are covered by the government for psychotherapy but don't offer it. This leaves the task to clinical psychologists and other mental health professionals. But the government does not pay for it. If patients have any coverage, it is a benefit from their employers. But most of these policies only cover six sessions – a length that research has long shown to be inadequate (Howard et al., 1986). Even this brief number of sessions may not be available unless you work for a large company that can afford to be generous. (This may explain why in recent years I have evaluated many baristas from Starbucks.)

Current data suggest that most patients benefit from a defined weekly course of sessions with specific targets, *but that those with severe problems need more* (Nordmo et al., 2021). But there are hardly any clinical trials supporting therapies that last more than 12 months. Admittedly, longer therapies are more difficult to study, but should we prescribe them in the absence of empirical support?

After a century of open-ended treatments, we have no evidence that *any* psychotherapy needs to go on for years. The few comparisons that have been made between shorter and longer courses of treatment have found *no* difference in outcome (Juul et al., 2023; McMain et al., 2022). Moreover, long-term psychotherapy may have compromised the credibility of this treatment. Advocates have argued that clinical trials of extended open-ended therapy are rare because they are too expensive. For this reason, some have devoted their careers to studying the process of therapy rather than its outcome.

Biological psychiatrists (e.g., Taylor, 2013) dismiss talking therapies as well meaning but ineffective. Their conclusions are not well informed. Most psychiatrists do not regularly read journals or know much about the science behind psychological treatment. Thus, a great divide between biology and psychology remains in place in psychiatry, which can be seen as a kind of dualism (Miresco and Kirmayer, 2006). If more clinicians were familiar with the research literature, they might embrace a broader and more eclectic practice.

7.2 Psychotherapy Is Usually Effective

Research has found psychotherapy to be efficacious for a wide variety of problems. That conclusion was supported decades ago by the first meta-analyses (Smith et al., 1980), and research up to the present has consistently confirmed it (Cuijpers, 2024). There is also good evidence that psychotherapy can produce measurable changes in the brain (Barsaglini et al., 2014).

Thus, the status of psychotherapy as evidence-based treatment is as strong as for most of the medications that we prescribe. About two-thirds of depressed patients who receive psychological treatment achieve a symptomatic remission, which is about the same percentage as for antidepressants. Although that is not a very high bar, it compares well to other areas of medicine. Why are we not helping a larger number? We need to improve our methods to achieve more consistent results. Evidence-based therapies have a good track record, but too many practitioners offer methods that lack evidence, and/or offer support without structure. Thus, psychotherapy is all too often unstandardized and not sufficiently accountable.

Keep in mind that not every patient responds to even the most skilled therapies. There could be many reasons: disorders that are not suitable for standard interventions, therapists who offer the same package to all their clients, or patients who reject therapy because they do not see how "just talking" could help. Even so, research shows that depressed patients have a more stable long-term outcome after therapy than those who receive medication alone (Cuijpers, 2024).

7.3 Poor Access to Good Therapy

Many psychotherapies are evidence-based, but access to them is problematic. Patients who could benefit from psychological interventions may never be offered the option. Even when psychiatrists carry out consultations and recommend psychotherapy, they may not be able to find a good clinician – unless the patient or the family is wealthy. Fees for the best-trained providers are out of range for most patients. Typically, the current cost of a weekly therapy session is about $150–$200 in the USA, and about £60–£100 in the UK. Insurance covers a minimal length of treatment. Publicly funded therapy is hard to find, and waiting lists are common.

Where I work, psychotherapy is only funded by the government in community clinics staffed with a limited number of psychologists. Moreover, patients usually have to wait months before starting treatment. In practice, some psychologists offer psychotherapy on a sliding scale. Even though research shows that low frequencies of sessions are less effective (Erekson et al., 2015), patients may have to come only once every two weeks to afford the fees.

While most psychiatrists receive training in psychotherapy, the system does not encourage them to make it part of their normal practice, and only a minority know how to use these skills to yield substantial change. When medication is the only treatment, it falls within the "15-minute hour," leaving little time for discussion. The most frequent pattern is to split the treatment. Thus, psychologists or other nonmedical clinicians provide psychotherapy, and if medication is needed, most patients receive that treatment from primary care doctors (or, less often, from psychiatrists, internists, or nurse practitioners). Split treatments make the main role of psychiatrists to be a consultant to other professionals.

One disadvantage of this model is that a prescriber can be locked into renewing or adjusting medications, but not to discontinue drugs when they are ineffective or no longer needed. Psychiatrists are not well trained on how to stop medication and are more likely to renew a current regime or select an alternative pharmacological option. It could be said we know how to add but not how to subtract.

The result is that patients end up taking too many medications for too long. Given the common (but incorrect) belief that all depressions require antidepressants, focusing on pharmacotherapy becomes almost unavoidable. While there is evidence that patients with recurrent depressions benefit from long-term prophylaxis (Looi et al., 2025), it is hard to separate them from those who do not need to keep taking antidepressants.

Where I work, access to psychiatric consultation is fully insured by the government, but there is a waiting list of several months before patients can be seen, and another wait for treatment when available. That is why the emergency room (ER) – or as it is called in the UK, accident and emergency (A&E) – is a major point of entry to the mental health system. But if you go to the ER, you will have to sit for hours before being evaluated. Then, if treatment is not deemed to be an emergency, you will be put on a waiting list for follow-up. Clinics that bridge these gaps are very rare. This lack of continuity leads psychiatrists in the ER to offer prescriptions to avoid sending patients away entirely untreated. But after that, there may be no one to follow up on medications or deal with side effects.

Access to psychotherapy can be increased by offering it online (Galvin et al., 2022), in which case fees are usually reduced. One recent survey found that the use of teletherapy has increased availability of this service, and that more patients are receiving it (Olfson et al., 2024). Even so, patients or their families still have to pay for the treatment.

Finally, the population has had an increase in "mental health literacy" (Bonabi et al., 2016). For this reason, we see an increased demand for mental health treatment – but in the absence of any increase in accessibility. The situation may be worse in countries where psychological treatment of sufficient length and frequency is not covered by insurance. Companies that cover mental health treatment are fearful of having to pay out for years instead of months. Their concern is by no means irrational, since therapies have some tendency to go on for indefinite periods of time. But given that most insurance plans pay for chronic physical illness, limitations on mental health coverage are an example of stigma. This lack of parity derives from a negative attitude to mental illness. No physician would treat diabetes or kidney failure within a strict time limit.

The prospects for broader access are somewhat better in the UK. A program called *Improving Access to Psychological Therapies* (IAPT, now known as NHS Talking Therapies) was set up within the National Health Service. It offers cognitive therapy for anxiety and depression. But IAPT does not, however, cover therapy for more severe forms of psychopathology. Moreover, the National Health Service has been suffering from budget cuts that make its system less of a model for other countries. Germany has long had the most comprehensive coverage (Altmann et al., 2016), but even in developed countries, access remains problematic.

One of the main reasons for promoting better insurance is that psychotherapy is *cost-effective* (Lazar, 2010). Patients receiving psychological treatment get back to work faster. Without therapy, all too many stop working and collect disability payments over many months or longer (supported by forms filled out by well-meaning physicians). The longer disability payments go on, the less likely patients are to return to the workforce (Marrone and Golowka, 1999). This policy is clearly counterproductive. The cost of treatment is much less to society than putting patients on disability.

My view, based on research findings, is that if governments or private insurance were willing to insure 20 sessions a year of psychotherapy for all citizens, sick leaves would be shorter, patients would go back to work, and insurers would actually *save* money (Smith et al., 2025).

7.4 Psychotherapy Should Usually Be Brief

Therapy has a beginning, but all too often lacks an ending. There is always something to talk about. And if you have the money or the insurance, why give up a relationship with a wise and trusted confidante? That scenario is all too common.

But how did it happen that therapy began to go on for *years*? Freud started out by offering a few months of daily meetings. When that framework did not accomplish what he expected, he extended the length of treatment, but eventually acknowledged there was something "interminable" about his method (Freud, 1937/1962).

Too many therapists since that time have fallen into the same trap. Trainees are still being taught to believe that therapy *should* take years, on the grounds that if problems have lasted for years, treatment should also go on for years. That is hardly an evidence-based point of view. What research shows is that most therapies need only last for a few months, and that they rarely need to be longer. Again, in spite of half a century of research, there is *no* evidence to support continuing therapy for more than 6–12 months.

There is strong evidence, however, showing that brief therapy (up to about 20 sessions) is efficacious for a majority of patients. That framework also applies both to cognitive therapy, as well as to short-term psychodynamic therapies (Abbass et al., 2012). Moreover, direct comparisons between longer and shorter lengths of therapy almost always show identical results. This is why I think that every therapy should have a time limit. We need to plan discharge from the beginning and encourage patients to become their own therapist.

I have wrestled with these problems since the beginning of my career. When I founded specialized clinics for patients with BPD 25 years ago, it was based on concern about access to care. I often saw patients who were receiving only what psychotherapy researchers call "treatment as usual," that is, the usual mess of follow-up for troubled patients in clinics. I first encountered these patients working in a student health clinic, where I could offer several months of therapy. University students, whose treatment was covered by insurance, were among the few patients who had rapid access to therapy without breaking the bank.

As discussed in Chapter 4, about 25 years ago, I founded a program for BPD in a general hospital where the burden of suicidal patients in the ER was a major problem. There are now similar programs at other hospitals in the city. We have documented that most patients could be successfully treated within 3 months, and that those who needed more than that could be managed within 6 or at the most 12 months (Laporte et al., 2018). Our approach could be described as "DBT lite" – building on the ideas of Linehan (1993) by teaching skills for managing emotional dysregulation.

Effectiveness data on 479 patients supported these impressions, with about two-thirds of BPD showing symptomatic recovery (Laporte et al., 2018). Our patients did not necessarily reach full remission on discharge but were well on the road to recovery. As Zanarini (2018) found in a 24-year follow-up, once patients are on a track to recovery, they continue to improve over time.

If you work with patients who are severely dysfunctional, you will have some failures. But we were satisfied with what we could accomplish for the majority. Our rate of symptomatic remission was about the same as in psychotherapy as a whole, or with medication by itself. And only 12% percent of patients came back asking for more therapy.

We are not the only ones to offer time-limited treatment for BPD. In Canada, the health system is insured by the provinces, and it allows clinicians working in hospitals to offer specialized time-limited therapy. A university-sponsored clinic in Toronto conducted a comparison of 6 vs. 12 months of dialectical behavior therapy – and found no difference in outcome (McMain et al., 2022). In the USA, the University of Iowa developed a well-structured program of brief group therapy, called STEPPS (Systems Training for Emotional Predictability and Problem Solving) that has been tested in several clinical trials with positive outcomes (Blum and Black, 2020). Brief targeted courses of treatment are, in my view, the future of psychotherapy, even in patients with severe personality disorders.

7.5 Common Factors: How Therapy Works

There are hundreds of brand name psychotherapies on the market today. How should clinicians choose among them?

A large body of research supports the conclusion that psychotherapy is effective for a wide range of psychological problems. But it also finds few differences in outcome between methods based on different theories or specific interventions. There is little reason to choose among most forms of treatment, each with its own three-letter or four-letter acronym. This finding supports the idea that *common factors* are more important for outcomes than interventions associated with specific methods. If most therapies do much the same thing, their efficacy must at least in part be related to what they share.

What are these common factors? As shown by meta-analyses (Norcross and Lambert, 2019; Wampold and Imel, 2015), the strength of the relationship to the therapist seems to be the more important factor. Successful clinicians, no matter what their training, have an unusual ability to empathize with patients. Above all, a sense of connection and trust can drive therapy forward and support both emotional and behavioral change. And what patients remember most about their therapy is the feeling of being understood (Strupp et al., 1969).

Yet while empathy is a necessary condition for therapy, it is not sufficient. We can go back many decades to the work of Carl Rogers (1995), who described the basic conditions for good treatment as **unconditional positive regard, empathy, and congruence (i.e., authenticity)**. These Rogerian methods, called "client-centered psychotherapy," were supported by a small body of research, but are less used today in their original form. Perhaps this system is best suited to people without severe psychopathology. I have seen too many patients whose previous therapies failed because the patient was offered empathy – but little in the way of explanation or guidance.

Therapists need to teach patients *skills* that promote change. This means clinicians need to be active, not silent, or only offering "interpretations." Once a therapeutic alliance is established, they should not be afraid of giving advice, which is more likely to be followed once trust is established. That is one of the secrets behind the success of cognitive behavioral therapy (CBT). This method, now considered standard, aims to change the way patients think. But it does more than that. CBT therapists can spotlight dysfunctional behaviors that are not working for the patient's goals. They should also not be shy about making tactful suggestions for trying out new behaviors. Doing so helps avoid the stagnation that comes from limiting the discussion to weekly life events.

7.6 Too Many Therapies, Too Little Integration

Psychotherapy has suffered from the promotion of too many models. Research has consistently shown that the efficacy of therapies is about the same for all evidence-based methods. Again, meta-analyses show that the name of a therapy and its technical toolkit are not as important to outcome as the skill of therapists in establishing a relationship (Norcross and Karpiak, 2024; Wampold and Imel, 2015). Therefore, we should be doing more research on the skills of care providers and less on the theories that underlie many brands of therapy. We now have hundreds of them, each claiming to be different, in spite of the fact that they all do much the same thing.

In summary, too much emphasis has been given to therapies that claim to be unique but are not actually new. That is why head-to-head comparisons between well-structured therapies do not find differences in outcomes. What counts is the use of a relationship that combines understanding emotions with guiding patients to adopt better coping skills (Norcross and Karpiak, 2024).

The rise of evidence-based medicine, in which randomized clinical trials (RCTs) are required to support treatment recommendations, has changed the landscape for the treatment of physical and mental illnesses (Sackett et al., 1996). And given the replication crisis in medicine and psychology, one RCT is never enough. It is best to wait until a meta-analysis of multiple trials can be carried out. That is the framework used by Cochrane reports, which have done so much to support evidence-based practice (EBP; Barbui et al., 2017). Similar requirements for research are required in order to be listed as evidence-based by the American Psychological Association (Spring, 2007).

Unfortunately, psychoanalysis put psychiatry and clinical psychology on the wrong track. To be fair, Freud lived in an era when evidence-based medicine of any kind lay far in the future. But his claim to scientific status for his methods, at least in their initial form, was dubious. When therapy does not work, the treatment could go on for years in the absence of evidence to support doing so (Smit et al., 2012). As noted earlier, there is also evidence from meta-analyses that brief targeted therapy based on psychodynamic principles yields about the same outcomes as CBT (Abbass et al., 2012).

When I was a resident, we were taught "eminence-based" rather than evidence-based therapy. This point of view was especially notable among psychiatrists who had additional training in psychoanalysis, a domain where research was not part of the curriculum. But clinical experience alone should not guide us; it has been described as "making the same mistakes with increasing confidence over an impressive number of years" (O'Donnell, 1997). Or, to quote an oft-quoted aphorism, the plural of anecdote is not data.

Even in Freud's time, psychoanalytical ideas were seen as fanciful by academic psychiatrists. He was also challenged by defectors from his movement who preferred their own ideas to those of a self-declared authority. This led to a free-for-all, allowing every therapist to come up with their own method. That scenario is what all too often happens. And it still does.

When I trained in psychiatry, the alternatives to psychodynamic therapy were not attractive. Behavior therapy denied any role for the mind, while Rogerian therapy assumed that patients could improve on their own with minimal interventions. Moreover, biological psychiatry was more interested in medication than talking therapy of any kind.

A turning point came with the introduction of CBT (Beck and Haigh, 2014). Beck, originally trained as a psychoanalyst, developed a model that aimed to change the way people think about and process life problems. His group was among the first to conduct RCTs that found CBT to be efficacious for anxiety and depression. The length of therapy was generally 20 sessions – just a few months (instead of the years psychoanalysts believed were necessary). Brevity made therapy affordable for many people. But the question remains as to whether the success of CBT is due to its theory, or to having a structured and active approach to the problems for which patients seek help. It also focuses collaboration, pioneering shared evaluations of results with patients. This having been said, there is no evidence from large meta-analyses that CBT produces consistently better results than its competitors (Cuijpers et al., 2023).

The centrality of common factors has led many psychotherapy researchers to advocate for an integrated model (Norcross and Karpiak, 2024). This approach is most consistent with the evidence, so one might have expected it to dominate the field. But that is not what happened. While CBT is considered standard, newer methods continued to fascinate clinicians not satisfied with limited efficacy. With acronyms in hand, newer models are marketed through courses, seminars, and books. Quite a few are "trauma-focused" (Jericho et al., 2022), a niche based on a currently hot topic. But the efficacy of these newer therapies is no better than for classical CBT (Paris, 2024).

Several of these newer methods are part of a group of "third wave" therapies that derive from CBT but focus more on managing emotions than on cognitive reframing. One of the most influential is dialectical behavior therapy (DBT; Linehan, 1993), originally developed for suicidal patients with personality disorders such as BPD, but also used for addictions (Haktanır and Callender, 2020). DBT applies an eclectic mix of ideas, many of which are both original and effective. One principle that I have found particularly useful is "radical acceptance." Here, in contrast to trauma-focused therapies and psychoanalysis, patients are encouraged to put their past behind them and to move on to a better future that they can be helped to create.

The most important contribution of DBT concerns the teaching of skills to promote emotion regulation. Theories about how we process emotions have stimulated a good deal of research (Gross, 2015). With these studies in mind, Barlow et al. (2020) proposed a *unified protocol* for managing high levels of trait neuroticism. This "transdiagnostic" approach cuts across disorder categories, which tend to be comorbid, including anxiety disorders, depression, PTSD, as well as personality disorders associated with emotion dysregulation.

7.7 Psychotherapy: The Missing Piece of Psychiatric Practice

This book has argued that a biopsychosocial theory of mental disorders requires biopsychosocial treatment. Yet few psychiatrists today offer formal psychotherapy that are applications of a large body of psychological research. One obstacle is beliefs about the causes of psychopathology. In a survey of mental health clinicians, those who espoused a primarily biomedical model were found to be less empathic than those who believed that life experience also plays a major role in psychopathology (Lebowitz and Ahn, 2014).

There are still psychiatrists who do nothing except psychotherapy. But I do not recommend that kind of practice. First of all, it wastes years of medical training, since the same treatment can be carried out by other professionals. Second, if there is generous insurance of coverage for physicians (as in Canada), therapy can be interminable. A survey in Toronto found that a subgroup of office-based psychiatrists rarely saw new patients, mostly because they held on to the old ones (Kurdyak et al., 2014). The treatments they did offer were not evidence-based, but supportive open-ended therapy combined with prescriptions (Gratzer and Goldbloom, 2016).

I also do not see any likelihood of getting psychiatrists to offer a larger amount of psychotherapy in practice. I did so in my own career only because I subspecialized in BPD, a condition for which medication is not very helpful, and for which psychotherapy is strongly indicated. Providing psychotherapy should be part of the armamentarium of psychiatrists who treat disorders that respond best to it – that is, addictions, eating disorders, and personality disorders. Empathic skills engender trust and may also benefit treatment that is mainly biological.

Psychiatrists are a key link in the process of mental health consultation. That is where referrals to psychotherapy should usually be generated. But we need to get past the obstacle of access and cost. If governmental health insurance covered a reasonable number of evidence-based sessions a year, that might well do the trick. The main reason that has not happened is the stigma of mental illness, which allows insurers, both public and private, to believe that mental illnesses that are not psychotic are not real, but just an excuse for not working.

Answer to Unanswered Question #7
Psychotherapy is both effective and cost-effective. Psychiatrists should offer this option if they treat the disorders that have been shown to respond to it. But only some practice in that way, and if they do offer talking therapy, it may not be evidence-based. Most of the providers are clinical psychologists who are rarely well insured. These restrictions are not quite rational, but reflect the continuing stigma associated with mental disorders.

Chapter

8 Suicide

Unanswered Question #8: Why, in spite of extensive research, are psychiatrists unable to predict or prevent suicide?

8.1 Why Clinicians Cannot Predict or Prevent Suicide

Suicide is an emotional tragedy. When fatalities occur, they damage survivors and seriously affect mental health clinicians (Sandford et al., 2021). Yet past surveys have found that at least half of mental health practitioners will lose a patient by suicide in the course of their career (Chemtob et al., 1988). If psychiatrists have not had that experience, they may have either run a very small practice or restricted it to patients who are not severely ill.

I have written a book, now in a second edition, about patients with *chronic* suicidality (Paris, 2023b). Let me summarize and update those conclusions here. This chapter could have been titled "myths of suicide prevention." In spite of decades of research, we do not know how to prevent people from dying by suicide. Yet almost every article published in scientific journals concerning suicidality tells its readers that research can be applied to prevention.

What is the evidence that psychiatrists or psychologists actually have the means to prevent fatal outcomes? The short answer is that there isn't any. What we can do is to prevent further attempts in patients who have tried to kill themselves. That is a different question entirely.

The explanation for this paradox is simpler than you think. Suicide is rare (affecting about 10–13/100,000 of the US population). Suicide attempts are much more common, at nearly 5% of the population over a lifetime, while the lifetime prevalence of suicidal ideation is even higher, close to 14% of the population (Kessler et al., 1994). It is difficult if not impossible to predict a rare event from a common one. The vast majority of those who think of suicide or attempt it will not die by their own hand.

There are two populations of patients with suicidality. One consists mainly of males who tend not to seek help, whose method is firearms or hanging, and who die on their first attempt. These patients are only a minority of those seen by psychiatrists. The second group is mainly female, highly help-seeking, with suicide attempts that are typically overdoses of pills. These are the patients who present most often in emergency settings, where they may be held over for observation to prevent suicide. But long-term follow-up studies show that the eventual suicide rate in this population is only 3%.

The problem is that attempters cannot be distinguished from those who eventually kill themselves (Paris, 2023b). This means that most suicide attempts are *false positives* for fatality. Psychiatrists are asked to evaluate the risk for suicide in individual patients, even though there is no evidence that they can reliably do so. Treating these cases may prevent additional attempts, but not fatalities.

Is there a scientific way of predicting suicide risk? The answer again is no. While psychiatrists and their students are expected to use risk factors to guide assessment, none consistently predict fatality. Some believe they can use a list of statistically derived risk factors to make predictions. But as we will see, applying these algorithms are no better than guessing.

Decades ago, two large-scale studies used multiple risk factors such as age, diagnosis, method of attempt, number of prior attempts, suicidal ideation on admission, outcome at discharge, level of social support, and a family history of mania, to predict suicide after an admission to a hospital for suicidality. In the largest study of 5,412 formerly hospitalized psychiatric patients in Iowa, 68 died by suicide. That rate (1.3%) is higher than we find in the general population. Even so, the vast majority did not kill themselves. And given that all were hospitalized, this was a high-risk population. Accidental deaths accounted for another minority of cases (0.7%).

In another prospective study, 4,800 hospitalized veterans were followed for a mean of five years. Predictions of fatal outcomes were made using a similar list of risk factors to the Iowa study. Again, most cases were false positives, with only 67 patients dying by suicide. In both of these studies, there was a statistical relationship between the risk algorithms and a fatal outcome, but the number of false positives was too high to identify individual cases.

Both were pioneering studies. Unfortunately, while decades have passed since their publication, only a few further large-scale prospective studies of suicide prediction among attempters have been carried out. In several cases, (De Moore and Robertson, 1996; Powell et al., 2000), the number of false positives was again too high to predict fatalities. A large registry study of nearly 40,000 attempters in Sweden after at least 20 years (Tidemalm et al., 2008) found that the majority of deaths by suicide were related to schizophrenia or bipolar illness, but false positives were frequent. A Finnish study that followed over 1,000 attempters, most of whom were men, for 14 years (Suokas et al., 2001) found a fatality rate of 6.7%, but again, risk factors were not sufficiently robust to make any predictions concerning the patients who eventually died by suicide. A British follow-up over an average of 11 years of almost 13,000 patients who came to emergency for suicide attempts (Zahl and Hawton, 2004) found that only 3% eventually killed themselves.

More recently, it has been proposed that due to its ability to consider interactions between multiple risk factors, artificial intelligence (AI) monitoring suicidal ideation could be used to predict suicide (Kessler et al., 2020). At this point, no data show that AI can usefully anticipate fatalities. There is also no strong evidence that this technology can prevent further attempts (Pigoni et al., 2024; Walsh et al., 2017).

All these findings make most sense in the context of there being two partially overlapping suicidal populations in clinical practice. The highest risk for fatality lies in men who are not seen in psychiatry and is much lower in the women we most frequently evaluate.

If suicide cannot be predicted in individual cases, clinical interventions alone are unlikely to make it preventable. Based on the current state of evidence is that we should treat the problems that make patients consider suicide and not be distracted by a fear of what we cannot prevent.

Even if we cannot prevent death by suicide, good evidence shows that patients with suicidal ideation and/or attempts can be treatable as outpatients, using psychotherapy to manage their symptoms (Turecki et al., 2019). What research shows is that rapidly accessible treatments for suicidality lower the rate of nonfatal *attempts*. Doing so does not constitute suicide *prevention*. Rather, suicidal behaviors reflect severe distress, which is accompanied by ambivalence about dying, prompting a kind of Russian roulette of behaviors.

8.2 The Problem of Chronic Suicidality

I have long been interested in patients who suffer from suicidal ideation and make attempts over many years. My book on chronic suicidality (Paris, 2023b) quotes the poet Keats by being titled *Half in Love with Death*, with emphasis on the word *half*.

Many patients who make suicide attempts are admitted to psychiatry on the grounds of promoting "safety." But there is an absence of evidence that hospitalization can prevent fatal outcomes in *chronically* suicidal patients. This is a unique clinical scenario. Admission has a clear rationale for severe melancholic depression, which responds to biological treatments that save lives. But chronic suicidality is a very different problem. These patients often meet criteria for borderline personality disorder.

There are no treatments for this population that requires admission to a psychiatry ward. Sometimes patients are admitted briefly, not to prevent another attempt but to review the situation and to make a treatment plan. That option might be useful for patients who take large overdoses and/or require intensive medical care. But only a minority of attempters need to be in hospital; most express their ambivalence by calling someone for help. For this reason, patients who attempt suicide can benefit most from a timely crisis intervention that includes psychotherapy.

Where I work, clinical psychologists are expected to follow a guideline that requires them to send *all* patients with suicidal ideation to an emergency setting. This is a well-meaning but highly counterproductive rule. Most psychiatrists in an ER will not admit these patients to hospital, where the wards are already overcrowded, but may observe them in an overnight hold to collect more information. Even if clinicians were to follow this guideline, it would not prevent a single suicide. What it would do is to make chaotic ERs even worse places for chronically suicidal patients to visit. If these patients are admitted, they will not receive active treatment and may even be harmed by the experience.

But when patients have nowhere else to go, they may go to the emergency room. The frequency of suicide attempts and self-harm as presenting symptoms in that setting has greatly increased in recent decades (Bommersbach et al., 2024). While those who present with suicidality in ER eventually have a higher rate of death by suicide (Olfson et al., 2021), keep in mind that prospective research shows they are a small minority, and that we do not know which patients are most at risk (Hawton, 2014).

Some of the other approaches to suicidality that have been researched are more subtle. They include encouraging family doctors to be alert to the possibility of suicide, contacting people in the patient's social network, or simply sending a series of cards in the mail stating that the treatment team remains interested in the patient's case. But all this research suffers from small samples and uncertain generalizability. As discussed in Chapter 5, medications for specific mental disorders (clozapine for schizophrenia, lithium for bipolarity) can lower suicide rates, but do not eliminate the risk.

8.3 Population-Based Suicide Prevention

The most evidence-based methods of suicide prevention are not clinical interventions but interventions at a population level. That mainly requires reducing access to means. Since men tend to kill themselves with firearms, gun control could make a difference. But we lack the data (not to speak of the political will) to support such a program. The gun culture in countries like the USA is powerful. Even so, there are cultural factors – Canada places few restrictions on gun ownership but has a lower rate of suicide (Varin et al., 2021).

There is also evidence that placing barriers on bridges can prevent suicide in those who are ambivalent about dying (Atkins Whitmer and Woods, 2013; Okolie et al., 2020; Sinyor et al., 2024). In an article based on interviews with people who jumped off the Golden Gate Bridge in California but survived, a majority reported that they regretted their decision half the way down (Seiden, 1978).

Suicide rates vary a good deal across the globe. That suggests that suicide has strong social determinants, as has been known for more than a century (Durkheim, 1979/1897; Mueller et al., 2021). Rates in the USA have gone up in recent years (Martínez-Alés et al., 2022), but not in Canada (Varin et al., 2021). Most European countries have lower rates than the USA (Naghavi, 2019). Some developing countries (e.g., the African nation of Lesotho) have unusually high rates associated with social disintegration and a high prevalence of alcoholism, but other developing countries (e.g., Jamaica) have fairly low rates (Naghavi, 2019).

There always have been and will always be suicides. You can even read about them in the Bible. My view is that we are doing a good job of managing patients who attempt or threaten suicide. We have psychotherapy tools that are known to be effective. Just don't call it prevention.

Paradoxically, this is the plus side of our inability to predict suicide. First, a clear majority of patients who consider or attempt suicide are looking for reasons to live – which is why they seek therapy. Many of those who overdose tell a friend what they have done, a scenario usually ending in an ER visit. Second, we have the choice of a number of evidence-based methods that have been shown to reduce suicidal behaviors, as a Cochrane report found in its review of treatment for BPD.

Note, however, that self-harm, usually by cutting, is *not* suicidal behavior. That is why it is called non-suicidal self-injury (NSSI). Rather it is a way, that can eventually become addictive, to blunt dysregulated emotions by replacing psychological distress with physical pain (Linehan, 1993). Some patients who self-harm may go on to take overdoses (Turecki et al., 2019), but attempts do not reliably predict death by suicide.

8.4 Suicidal Patients with Personality Disorders

I have focused much of my career on BPD, motivated by the challenge of chronic suicidality. I could never be sure how much I was helping patients, but if they ended by giving up the option of death, something may have gone right.

What I long failed to understand was that 95% of these patients would never have died by suicide, with or without treatment. We found a 10% suicide rate in our 27-year follow-up of BPD cases. But since this population did not receive evidence-based treatment, we remain unsure as to whether therapy would have prevented suicide. Since starting specialized programs over the last 25 years, we found that of the first 1,000 patients treated in our clinics, only 5 died of suicide. We have not conducted a long-term follow-up on this cohort, but a better estimate of fatality comes from longitudinal studies of patients evaluated in emergency settings, with a fatality rate closer to 3%. But these numbers are too small for prediction. In retrospect, the deck was stacked in our favor. The data from our follow-up research made me less fearful: Even if 10% end up dying by their own hand, the most common outcome was that by a mean age of 50, over 90% of patients eventually chose to go on living (Paris and Zweig-Frank, 2001).

I remain cautiously optimistic about treating suicidal patients, but my approach has changed over the years. I finished my training in 1972, when many of my teachers were psychoanalysts. In spite of doubts, I followed this model in the early years of my career. It was interesting and illuminating to explore life stories, but it soon became obvious that significant change requires learning to make better choices in the present. I also concluded that therapies that go on for too long lead to repetition and stasis. Here it helped to have been trained in short-term treatment, working within a predetermined and motivating time limit. I also benefited from working part-time at a university health service, where students had more reasons to go on living.

When I was treating suicidal patients, my treatments went on for longer. I no longer see doing so as necessary. I was not yet converted to evidence-based practice or reading Cochrane reports. But what were the alternatives? Most methods of therapy are designed for less severe cases of anxiety and depression.

Then came dialectical behavior therapy (DBT), the first therapy for suicidality to be tested and found to be efficacious in a randomized clinical trial (Linehan, 1993). I admire Linehan, who has contributed so much to the management of these patients. But DBT is too long and too expensive for most patients. Its cost (tens of thousands of dollars) makes treatment unavailable for the patients who need it most. The method has also never been tested for more than a year but can go on longer. In the USA, insurance for extended treatments is limited. In the UK, DBT is rarely offered by the National Health Service.

In Canada, hospitals groan under the weight of patients who attempt suicide but are not easily managed in therapy. Thus, with a team of four senior clinicians, including another psychiatrist, a CBT psychologist, and a forensic psychologist, we opened a clinic 25 years ago to treat patients with 12 weeks of individual and group therapy. All had to meet diagnostic criteria for BPD. We now have a larger team (about 12, including trainees), as well as clinics and that offer 6–12 months of therapy.

All these programs can be considered as "DBT lite," as they include a blend of ideas from other methods of therapy. Our effectiveness data have documented good outcomes, with a majority having significant symptomatic improvement, while only 12% of patients came back asking for more treatment (Laporte et al., 2018). Crucially, we ran these programs in the public sector, at large hospitals where therapy is paid for by the government. A brief course of treatment allowed us to treat up to 100 patients a year in the 12-week program. A combination of individual and group therapy is particularly applicable to this population, since emotion regulation skills can best be taught in groups.

Many were surprised at our ability to help patients in a brief time. But the idea that BPD patients must have years of therapy was never evidence-based. As noted in

Chapter 7, a similar DBT clinic in Toronto found no difference in the outcome of its program over 6 vs. 12 months (McMain et al., 2022). These findings are encouraging for the prospects of patients with chronic suicidality.

As discussed in Chapter 5, psychotherapy should be brief for most patients. That recommendation need not change, even for those who threaten suicide or attempt it. Some may need to return at a later point for another round of time-limited treatment. We offer that option in our clinic, where the initial length is usually 6 months, but patients are not allowed to exceed 18 months of therapy in total. Termination involves preparing patients to use learned skills to become their own therapists.

8.5 Prospects for the Management of Chronic Suicidality

In summary, psychiatrists have a unique role in managing suicidality. But not all mental health caregivers are comfortable with chronic suicidal ideas and repeated attempts. We may have no unique tools to offer, but the presence of a physician on a team reduces everyone's anxiety. It is easier to accept the fear that these patients evoke, if one knows that a few suicides are inevitable in clinical practice. A minority of patients can choose death over life, but we need not blame ourselves. Patients who are suicidal are usually looking for other options. In most cases, psychotherapy can help them find reasons for living.

Answer to Unanswered Question #8
Psychiatrists are currently unable to predict or prevent suicide. But they have an important role to play in treating patients who make suicide attempts or have suicidal ideation.

Chapter

9

Society

Unanswered Question #9: *Do psychiatrists have a mandate to recommend how modern society could be made less stressful?*

9.1 Social Risk Factors in a Biopsychosocial Context

Social psychiatry is concerned with the effects of social factors on the causes, course, and treatment of mental illness. Empirical evidence supports associations between social stressors and the frequency of mental disorders. Yet, like biological and psychological risk factors, these relationships are statistical, mainly applying to those with biological and/or psychological vulnerabilities. Once again, risks for psychopathology need to be framed within an interactive biopsychosocial model.

Research on social risks is largely based on the findings of *psychiatric epidemiology,* that is, differences in the prevalence of disorders in specific populations. Statistics are regularly collected on mental disorders and the patients who have them, and governments have supported large-scale surveys in many countries, especially Scandinavia and North America.

One recent survey in the USA estimated that 23% of the population meet the criteria for a mental disorder of some kind in any year (Reinert et al., 2024). That sounds like a major problem, but the number includes every category in the DSM. It is almost certainly an overestimate, and only 6% of the sample had a severe mental disorder. Of greater concern, only half of those with a mental disorder received treatment, mostly due to stigma and poor insurance coverage (Presskreischer et al., 2023). The percentage who received evidence-based treatments is undoubtedly lower. These obstacles, blocking access to effective treatment, will be discussed in Chapter 10.

9.2 Evidence for Social Risk in Mental Disorders

9.2.1 Socioeconomic Class

One of the best-known findings in psychiatric epidemiology is a higher prevalence of major mental disorders in the lower socioeconomic classes (Kivimaki et al., 2020). But as shown by a meta-analysis, it is a real (but small) effect. We could account for this finding in two ways. Socioeconomic deprivation can be a risk factor for mental disorders, but belonging to a lower class can be a consequence of having a disorder. Poverty is associated with many other risk factors, both at the individual and neighborhood levels.

9.2.2 Cross-Cultural Differences

The presence of cross-cultural differences in the prevalence of mental disorders provides the most convincing evidence for the role of social factors. Major mental disorders are found in all societies, but their prevalence is variable around the world (Eaton et al., 2008).

We can see the influence of culture more clearly when the prevalence of a disorder has been low in a population but increases when its members emigrate. For example, anorexia nervosa is rare in societies where there may not be enough to eat but becomes more common among emigrants from traditional to modern societies (DiNicola, 1990). With globalization, similar increases in the prevalence of eating disorders have been documented in countries where people may not emigrate – for example, in Fiji, a small island in the Pacific Ocean (Gerbasi et al., 2014).

Another source of evidence for social risk factors is that emigrants from Jamaica to the UK have a higher rate of psychosis than those who do not emigrate, an effect that has been attributed to "social defeat" in their new country (Selten and Cantor-Graae, 2007). These findings have been reported among minorities living in the UK, as well as in other European countries (Schalbroeck, 2023; Selten et al., 2020).

9.2.3 Cohort Effects

Changes in prevalence over time, or cohort effects, provide strong evidence for the presence of social factors in mental disorders. An increasing prevalence, in the same population and over a single generation, cannot be explained in any other way. Sometimes change is so rapid that it can be called *social contagion*. That process may be a factor in the recent increase of cases of self-harm in adolescents who imitate their peers (Paris, 2024). Although self-harm is not new, there is evidence that it is becoming more common as a way of controlling mental distress and dysregulated emotions.

9.2.4 Social Change and Social Cohesion

Emil Durkheim, one of the founders of sociology, is best known for a book on suicide (1979/1897), which showed that "anomie" (i.e., alienation) varied among religious groups and was associated with differences in rates of suicide. Another founder of sociology, Max Weber, examined some of the same questions when he described modern society as struggling with the effects of secularization and loss of religious faith, leading to a sense of isolation and disconnection (Whimster and Lash, 2014). We have not evolved to be alone in the world. Humans are highly social animals, which is probably the main reason for having a large "social brain" (Dunbar, 2009).

Sociological research consistently supports the idea that *social cohesion* is related to mental health (Friedkin, 2004). The same conclusion was made by the sociologist Pierre Bourdieu, who initiated the term *social capital* (Julien, 2015). These links to others have also been termed *social integration* (Turner and Turner, 1999). Whatever the terminology, we need stable connections that provide a sense of identity and belonging. When these supports are absent, we are more liable to develop mental disorders.

One of the major driving forces of social change in recent decades all over the world has been migration from rural areas to cities (Tacoli et al., 2015). But no evidence supports the romantic idea that life in the countryside is necessarily better than in a large city. There are no consistent urban–rural differences in the prevalence of mental disorders (Breslau et al., 2014). The tendency to idealize rural life has been called "the myth of paradise lost" (Srole and Fischer, 2021). People who live in rural areas can be just as lonely and socially isolated as those in crowded urban areas.

In recent decades, epidemiologists have been reporting a worldwide increase in depression (Moreno-Agostino et al., 2021). However, it is hard to know if this is a real change, a result of increased mental health literacy, or an artifact of measurement. Some studies, particularly in the USA, have found increases in suicidal ideation and attempts among younger adolescents (Bommersbach et al., 2024), although most of these are single episodes and do not usually become chronic (Bommersbach et al., 2025).

Assuming that an increase is real, the causes of increased depression could be an accelerating level of social change, especially a shift from a more collectivist society to one that rewards individualism (Markus and Kitayama, 2003). That shift in social values may also be a reason for documented increases in the prevalence of personality disorders (Paris, 2020c).

The rise of the internet can be another threat to social cohesion and has received a good deal of attention from researchers. One prominent social psychologist (Twenge, 2023) has proposed that the recent increase on depression among adolescents began in 2012, shortly after most owned an iPhone. One might think that having internet "friends" might be good for lonely people, but only up to a point. We have evolved to need real-life human connections, for which there is no substitute. The mechanism that ties excess time on the internet with depression could be that social media promotes social comparison, leading to feelings of incapacity (2024).

This raises the question as to whether adolescents in modern society are actually suffering from increases in rates of psychopathology or are only presenting more often to the mental health system. A recent longitudinal study in the UK of 3,000 adolescents failed to show that any major change has actually occurred (Plackett et al., 2023).

The social risk factors discussed previously do not affect a majority of the population. They interact with heritable vulnerabilities, as well as with differences in risk factors related to psychological environments. But social factors can be a "tipping point" for psychopathology. Thus, outcomes are usually related to cumulative risk, not to single variables.

For example, consider racial differences in psychopathology. Black populations in the USA face obstacles that can lead to social defeat and are more likely to grow up in single-parent families and in bad neighborhoods. But while this scenario sometimes leads to antisocial behavior, it need not. Extended families can make a difference – as shown by the life story of Barack Obama. In fact, blacks have long had a lower suicide rate than whites. The explanation may lie with higher social cohesion, often mediated by religious observance.

Now consider sex differences. Women in Western societies have faced many obstacles but have temperamental advantages. Females have evolved to benefit from social networks, whereas males are more likely to react to a loss of social status (Campbell, 2013). That helps explain some of the differences between men and women in the prevalence of mental disorders (Zahn-Waxler et al., 2015). Thus, most prisoners are men, most alcoholics are men, and the great majority of suicides occur in men. In contrast, more women suffer from depression, anxiety disorders, eating disorders, and from disorders associated with emotional dysregulation.

Social change can also be protective against psychopathology. Thus, when women who had participated in a major epidemiological study in New York City were followed 20 years later, their mental health had, on average, notably improved (Srole and Fischer, 2021). By and large, middle age is a better time than youth for most people. As much as mothers love their children, they have fewer symptoms when living in an "empty nest" (Romans and Seeman, 2006). Another factor is that now that more women are working outside the home, they have a separate source of satisfaction and self-esteem. These findings run contrary to the tendency to blame society for every aspect of modern unhappiness. We romanticize the past, but there is good reason to believe that for all the problems of modern life, we are living in one of the best times in human history (Pinker, 2011).

9.3 Should Psychiatrists Promote Social Change?

If social factors play an important role in the risk for mental disorders, should clinicians be promoting social change? I do not accept this view. Changing society does not lie within the mandate of either psychiatry or clinical psychology.

We need to ask whether there are any forms of social dysfunction that can, *by themselves*, be causes of mental disorders. Some have thought so. That view has been the position of "critical psychiatry," a movement that takes a skeptical view of drug treatments and that focuses on cross-cultural and cross-national differences in mental disorders (Kirmayer et al., 2015). I am sympathetic with many of the criticisms of mainstream practice that have been highlighted in social and transcultural psychiatry. In Canada, the most striking effects are seen in indigenous populations whose culture has been destroyed.

One might therefore think that mental disorders require an approach based on principles of public health. But we do not know enough to support that conclusion. Moreover, political change is not the province of medicine. The idea that social change can prevent psychopathology is a utopian ideological position that ignores the limitations of human nature. Programs based on radical social change have long been a recipe for failure.

Like other citizens, psychiatrists have a right to their political opinions. But that does not mean we should promote social change in the name of better mental health. Most practitioners, particularly academics, have left of center liberal views that lead them to adopt positions that favor central planning and a large role for government to protect the disadvantaged (Redding, 2023). But should these ideas be promoted by psychiatrists as a public health policy? I would also give this question a definite no. There is no Cochrane report for the efficacy of politic programs.

Finally, no one can accurately predict the future. Almost all attempts to make people happier and more functional by radically changing society (or its economic base) have come to grief and led to dystopias. Psychiatry is a medical specialty that needs to be based on empirical data. There is no evidence that we know more about how to run a society than members of any other profession. We are best advised to stick to our own expertise, which lies with individual patients. Unfortunately, if we are looking for answers about how to live our lives, we may be tempted to become pundits. The American Psychiatric Association has a "Goldwater rule" advising its members to avoid diagnosing people they have never met, especially politicians (Appelbaum, 2017).

9.4 Are Psychiatrists Experts in Parenting?

Parents are less sure today about how to raise their children – and may seek help from mental health professionals to get it right. As Furedi (2002) has pointed out, parents now lack confidence in their own judgments and are afraid of damaging their children. But there is no consensus about what is right and what is wrong. And experts don't necessarily agree with each other (Alwin, 2004). Moreover, parents are not alone, but are supported by extended family and social networks in what Hrdy (2009) calls "alloparenting."

Although I have worked most of my life with youth, I am not a child psychiatrist. Parenting my own children largely reflected the ideas of Benjamin Spock (1946), a pediatrician who had adopted psychoanalytic theory. Spock's ideas influenced a whole generation but have been seen as a force for "spoiling" children with too much empathy and not enough authority. That may be unfair, given Spock's consistent message that parents should trust their own judgment. But nothing in his book was based on research.

When I was in training, family therapy was a major focus in our university network. But psychiatrists, psychologists, and social workers applying this method did not carry out an evidence-based practice, and almost never quoted research when making recommendations. Their view was that children are "identified patients," and that pathology resides in the family system. This idea ignores most of what we now know about the role of temperament in children and how it impacts families.

To be fair, there is some evidence for the efficacy of family therapy, but it is by no means as voluminous as the data supporting individual psychotherapy. With time, family therapy has moved out of psychiatry and its leading figures are now mostly social workers.

Nonetheless, some psychologists – as well as people outside the mental health professions – continue to write books about how to raise children. I have no new ideas on this subject but am sympathetic to the view that we are suppressing healthy autonomy by overprotection and excessive worry about hurting the feelings of children (Haidt, 2024). On the other hand, I cannot agree with those, including a pediatrician at my university, who believe that there is such a thing as evidence-based parenting.

The problem is that much guidance by experts is rooted in cultural belief systems. Thus, our current rejection of strong parental authority is more about libertarian values than based on evidence about the best way of raising children. Other than the damage done by child abuse, I see few clear guidelines based on scientific data.

These observations have also affected what adult patients tell clinicians about their upbringing. Of course, patients are looking for explanations for their suffering. I was taught to make facile "formulations" about the effects of childhood experience based on these memories. But just about everyone has a story to tell about a bumpy childhood. Even the idea that a failure to validate emotions is central to the development of psychopathology is a half-truth. A child with a vulnerable temperament needs more validation than is the case for others. Every child is different, and each may require a somewhat different style of rearing.

9.5 Therapeutic Culture and Social Criticism

Social forces have affected psychiatry, but psychiatry has been an influential part of modernity. For this reason, our specialty, most particularly the practice of psychotherapy, has come under criticism. We are also criticized for having too much power over our patients. (If only that were true.)

One critique targets the development of a "therapeutic culture" that tells people how to live their lives and undermines the structure of families (Furedi, 2017). Psychotherapists have been accused of promoting narcissism by encouraging patients to privilege their psyche over the needs of others, leading to lower social cohesion (Lasch, 1978). Some psychologists (e.g., Baumeister, 2002) have gone so far as to suggest that the culture of talking therapy has replaced the role of religion in society.

None of these critiques applies to biological psychiatry, which is practiced in much the same way as general medicine. But psychiatrists who are involved with involuntary hospital admissions for patients with severe mental illnesses have been attacked for other reasons. Much of the criticism comes from a libertarian perspective, in which psychotic patients are seen as just having different ideas that they have the right to hold. Some of these critics argue against the use of medication in any form, even for patients who have been hospitalized (Szasz, 1960). But Szasz was successfully sued for discontinuing lithium on one of his patients – who then committed suicide after accepting that advice.

This is a story of how well-meaning ignorance has done damage not only to psychiatry but also to patients suffering from mental illnesses. When I began training at a large mental hospital, one of my teachers recommended reading a book by the French philosopher Michel Foucault. These ideas later became a major source for the "anti-psychiatry" movement (Foucault et al., 2013). The basic idea was that psychiatry is nothing but an abuse of power over people who are different. Along with sociologists (Scheff, 2017), some psychiatrists (Kirsner, 2015; Szasz, 1960), and one much-quoted (but fraudulent) psychologist (Rosenhan, 1973), these critics attacked psychiatry by denying that there was any such thing as mental illness. Of course, they could not explain why the human brain should differ from any other organ in the human body in its potential for dysfunction. All these critics did terrible damage to people suffering from severe mental disorders.

None of these critics (with the exception of Rosenhan) ever spent time in a psychiatric ward or an emergency room. One night in an ER might well have convinced them that our patients are ill, not just different. But the real agenda of the anti-psychiatry movement was shaped by the 1960s trend for opposing authority of any kind. Psychiatry became a target because of its power over involuntary civil commitment.

Since that time, I have been amazed at the adulation in social science and the humanities for Foucault's ideas. This man, one of the most cited writers of all time, was certainly a force of nature (Macey, 2019). But Foucault was no scientist, just a bad intellectual historian, making up narratives without evidence. Late in life, he was a supporter of the theocracy in Iran, and infected partners with the disease that eventually killed him. This "philosopher" had a way of covering his tracks – by denying the existence of objective reality in any domain. For Foucault, there was no objective truth, only power that is used to claim truth.

In the long run, the anti-psychiatry movement may have done mainstream practice a favor. Psychiatry gained respectability by adopting a research program designed to show that mental disorders are not essentially different from any other kind of illness. In any case, the mental hospitals of the past are gone, and hardly any psychotic patients wanted to be heroic rebels against society. These people were not necessarily cured, but most of them took their medication and were able to live in the community. Finally, many lives have been saved by psychiatry's ability to use civil commitment when patients are a danger to themselves or to other people (Appelbaum, 1992).

The reality of mental illness is clear when you see severe cases, which are common in emergency settings. The question of whether less severe problems should be diagnosed medically is a separate issue. The most sympathetic critics of psychiatry have warned against medicalizing normal life problems (Frances, 2013).

9.6 Prospects for Social Psychiatry

I have long been a supporter of social psychiatry, and have published a book on the subject (Paris, 2020c). But I worry that this domain has become too political. Some years ago, I raised this question with a colleague working with patients from other cultures. I was told, as often happens when you challenge someone's ideology, that my views were themselves politically motivated. Since we live in a multicultural society, we need to be critical of our assumptions. But for the followers of critical theory, there is no such thing as scientific neutrality.

Answer to Unanswered Question #9
Possessing knowledge of social risk factors is important for the clinical practice of psychiatry. But we are not trained to intervene on a societal level. We need to practice caution and humility and focus on the care of our patients.

Access to Mental Health Care

Unanswered Question #10: What can we do to increase access to mental health treatment?

10.1 Improving Access to Care

Psychiatry is far from being a panacea for mental illness. But its treatments are as effective as those offered by other physicians. Leucht et al. (2012) – reviewing 94 meta-analyses (48 for 20 medical diseases, and 16 for 8 mental disorders) – did not find superior efficacy in general medicine. Similar effect sizes have been documented by meta-analyses of the effectiveness of medication and psychotherapy in the treatment of depression (Cuijpers et al., 2022).

Even if the boundaries of specific mental disorders are unclear, psychopathology of some kind is ubiquitous. Depression ranks second for morbidity in most countries in the Global Burden of Disease research program (GBD Collaborators and Ärnlöv, 2020). As discussed in Chapter 9, these findings may not describe a true increase in prevalence. But mental health care has important things to offer and should be more easily available. Yet even in the most developed countries, people have difficulty accessing these services (Kazdin, 2018). But many of these disorders are never assessed or treated by professionals, whose services are not consistently covered by insurance (Coombs et al., 2021).

Kazdin (2018) has reviewed the most important obstacles to access in mental health care. The first is cost, the obvious but most important of these barriers. The second is that governments and third-party payers set restrictive conditions for how much treatment can be provided, and that mental health care is not given parity with physical illness. The third is that mental health professionals are too few to meet the needs of the population. Other obstacles have to do with attitudes. One is stigma, a second is low mental health literacy, and a third is cultural or ethnic discrimination.

The upshot is that some of the wealthiest countries have done little to make treatment more accessible, and, in many cases, have cut back on mental health services. For example, there are now fewer inpatient beds in hospitals. That might not be a problem if crisis intervention services were rapidly accessible. But they are either absent or weighed down by waiting lists. Where new services have been developed, they usually target less severe disorders (see discussion of the UK's IAPT program in Chapter 7). For more severe disorders affecting youth, early psychosis clinics have been shown to be cost-effective (Aceituno et al., 2019). But they are not matched by the availability of care for the chronically ill. Access is better in Australia, but even there, people who live in remote areas may not obtain it (Meadows et al., 2015). Germany ranks high in accessibility and does so by regulation of insurance companies, requiring that they cover mental disorders (Wiegand et al., 2025). Scandinavia is also a model for access and coverage (Wang et al., 2022).

One might think that a relative lack of access to mental health care would create strong public pressure for change. If patients on dialysis were not reimbursed for weekly treatments, there would be an uproar. But the patients who see psychiatrists and other mental health professionals rarely protest. Most do not even want anyone to know about their need for treatment. Since stigma is so powerful, only a few brave celebrities have "come out" with a story of their mental illness. Nor do care providers protest; they are busy, making a good living, and may not even perceive the extent of the problem.

Frances (2013) has pointed out that the large sums of money spent on neuroscience research have done little to help people with mental disorders, particularly the most severe ones. In Canada, the government has sometimes paid for large grants promoting access to care for the chronically ill. But their effects have been small. By and large, chronic mental disorders lack the priority that has been given to basic science. Surveys shed further light on these problems. For example, psychiatrists in the USA are less likely than other physicians to accept insurance (Bishop et al., 2014). Evidently, there are enough wealthy people to fill most practices.

One of the reasons I benefited from a career in Canada was the availability of comprehensive and universal health insurance. I never had to wrangle with managed care, as my American colleagues do. The Canadian system is underfunded but makes it easier to treat patients with limited resources, and to develop programs for patients with severe psychopathology. Moreover, physicians in publicly funded hospitals avoid burdensome paperwork by outsourcing to billing services. The most important difference in the Canadian system is that everyone has insurance, and that almost all psychiatrists accept it. The same applies to NHS-insured care in the UK. The main limitation, in both Canada and the USA, is that psychotherapy for more than a few sessions is not usually covered (even though, as discussed in Chapter 7, doing so for a few months a year would save the system money).

In spite of its commitment to universal health care, Canada has serious barriers to access (Moroz et al., 2020). Unlike the UK, 6 million Canadians (out of a population of 40 million) do not have a family doctor, and can remain on waiting lists for years before getting one. That is why hospital emergency rooms are crowded and dysfunctional. Technology cannot solve this problem. We need more professionals to provide care. Nurse practitioners have helped to some degree, but they are few, and most of their training is in psychopharmacology.

10.2 Can Online Treatment Address Problems of Access?

Like most psychiatrists, I provided online care to patients during the pandemic. Our personality disorder programs continued offering both group and individual therapy for emotion regulation skills during this time. But when the pandemic was over, most of us went back to seeing patients in our offices, only making exceptions for those who lived far from the hospital, or those who had work schedules that did not easily allow traveling.

Most of us prefer to see patients in person. But what does the evidence show? It suggests that virtual treatment is a reasonable option. Its delivery may not even require a professional. Cognitive Behavioral Therapy (CBT) offered virtually for the treatment of anxiety and depression is accepted by patients and yields about the same results (Gratzer and Goldbloom, 2016; Gratzer and Khalid-Khan, 2016). A meta-analysis of studies comparing in-person to online therapy came to the same conclusion, reporting an effect size of 0.53, which is about the same as in standard forms of practice. But not everyone agrees. An earlier review (Andersson and Titov, 2014) came to a different conclusion, expressing the concern that while online therapy is feasible, making diagnoses could be problematic when nonverbal phenomena are difficult to assess. (After the pandemic, I had trouble recognizing patients when they came in person to the hospital.) Nonetheless, a recent systematic review supported the overall effectiveness of telepsychiatry.

It is also likely that outcomes in virtual treatment vary depending on the severity of psychopathology; most studies have been conducted for CBT in common mental disorders, not for more disabling problems. But making online treatment available could be at least part of the answer to keeping some patients out of emergency. This kind of service delivery has been strongly recommended in Toronto, Canada, where there are more psychiatrists than elsewhere in the country, but where many practitioners rarely accept new patients, and do not necessarily take on those with severe mental disorders (Goldbloom, 2021).

10.3 Applying a Stepped-Care Model

Stepped care is a model of medical care in which patients initially receive brief and less intensive interventions and are only referred for longer and more intensive treatment when they do not respond to the first step (Bower and Gilbody, 2005). It aims to remove obstacles in the system by providing less care for patients who are likely to remit, and to offer more for those who are not. The model has been applied to depression (van Straten et al., 2015). An umbrella review of multiple meta-analyses (Jeitani et al., 2024) found stepped care to be superior to standard care for depression. It has also been used for more severe forms of psychopathology, such as BPD (Choi-Kain et al., 2016; Grenyer et al., 2018; Paris, 2017). One of its goals is to increase access for new patients.

I conclude that stepped care has great potential, but that more research will be needed before making it routine in practice. It could be a useful option for mental disorders that have a highly variable outcome. Its principles could encourage psychiatrists, in accordance with their medical training, to focus their efforts on the most difficult and complex patients.

10.4 Addressing Stigma

The difficulty of access to mental health treatment is a problem that thus far has been neither fully addressed nor solved. The gap between what surveys show about the prevalence of mental disorders and the percentage who access treatment remains large.

For one thing, the increase in demand for mental health services is not going away. There will never be enough psychiatrists to address this need, nor should there be. We need many more well-trained clinical psychologists, social workers, and occupational therapists. But they need to be insured, and that will cost money and serious investment by governments. The main reason that this has not happened is the stigma associated with having almost any kind of mental disorder.

The World Health Organization (2022) has made recommendations for reducing stigma and has published books on this subject (e.g., Rüsch, 2022). These ideas largely boil down to mental health awareness campaigns, with support from advocacy organizations. Many programs offer education and support for family members. A good example in the USA is the National Alliance on Mental Illness (NAMI; www.nami.org). There are similar organizations in the UK, such as Rethink Mental Illness (www.rethink.org/campaigns-and-policy/policy-and-influencing/stigma-and-discrimination/). A few celebrities have come forward about having been treated for mental symptoms, and some members of the UK royal family have done the same.

10.5 Prospects for Access to Care

The facts are that most people will either have an episode of mental illness over their lifetime or have had to cope with episodes in their family. These histories are not as stigmatized when symptoms are medical, but they tend to be when symptoms are psychiatric. Many still feel frightened about mental disorders and may withdraw trust and acceptance from those who suffer from them.

Meanwhile, patients are more likely to insure for surgery or for the cost of expensive medications than for prompt treatment of common mental disorders. But somehow the old idea of "getting a grip" is still alive and well, with the result that patients with mental symptoms may not be treated with the seriousness they deserve. These are long-term problems that require long-term solutions.

Answer to Unanswered Question #10
Lack of access to evidence-based mental health treatment may be the most serious problem in modern psychiatry. We need much more funding from governments, and we need psychiatrists to be more committed to the principles of accessibility.

Epilogue: A Prognosis for Psychiatry

E.1 Is Technology an Answer for Treating Mental Illness?

Predicting the future is all but impossible. That is why life is so full of surprises, with "black swan events" that have low probability but high impact (Taleb, 2007). Wars, famines, and epidemics almost always come unexpectedly.

We have long pinned hopes for the future on technology, a source of fascination and a driver of change. But breakthroughs are not necessarily a continuation of past advances. Hardly anyone predicted the key role of the internet before it was created.

Psychiatry changed radically when I was in training and during the early years of my career. The main reason was the availability of more effective psychopharmacology. Since then, in spite of further advances in neuroscience over the last half century, clinical work has not seen dramatic progress. Our medications have fewer side effects, but we do not know how they work or why they too often do not work. The same can be said about treatment with psychotherapy, in spite of large bodies of research (Markham et al., 2021).

We are waiting for breakthroughs, but they may not arrive in my lifetime or in the lifetime of my students. Even so, given the higher activity of research in psychiatry, it is hard to believe that the current stagnation of new treatments will continue indefinitely. The most important current question is whether neuroscience can eventually provide the tools to explain the causes of mental illness. But that requires knowing much more about the brain. It could well take many decades to solve the mysteries of the mind. Some preliminary work has been published linking symptoms to the findings of brain scans (Lett et al., 2025). But I am not convinced that we will find technological solutions any time soon to address all the complex problems that face psychiatry.

E.2 Is Artificial Intelligence an Answer?

Everyone these days is talking about AI. This term covers a wide range of projects (Kahn, 2024). Research is focusing on artificial general intelligence (when abilities of machines are better than those that humans have), and generative artificial intelligence (when AI offers new ideas beyond what can be obtained by machine learning).

AI is a tool for organizing large bodies of information. Its advantage is that it can deal rapidly with high levels of complexity. AI could easily provide clinicians with manualized diagnoses, as well as treatment options, without anyone having to look at DSM or ICD. But that is just a matter of convenience. A more important question is whether AI can develop a model of the brain connectome. Research on this technological fix has been at best preliminary, and its future in explaining mental illness remains uncertain (Shekouh et al., 2024).

Moreover, even if we were to use AI to make diagnoses, this advantage could turn out to be illusory, given that its input would have to be based on current diagnoses with uncertain validity. At this point, psychiatry's diagnostic systems remain sketchy and not very valid. Thus, as long as AI uses DSM or ICD diagnoses as dependent variables, doing so would only lead to a circularity that would not solve problems of classification. Machine learning might be better at seeing patterns in symptoms but it would still be limited by a lack of understanding of how the brain works. Some hope that dimensional diagnosis (as in RDoC and HiToP) would do better, but at this point, these systems offer little more than a way to account for "comorbidity."

What about using AI to guide treatment? The idea that AI can support a program of *personalized medicine* for psychiatric patients has been often proposed, but is premature (Maslej et al., 2023; Monteith et al., 2022). Personalized medicine makes sense when reading a genome helps physicians choose cancer treatments. But in spite of claims for pharmacogenetics, this model is not relevant to psychiatry – at least not yet. Using technology in this way is also not consistent with what we now know about genomic variations in major mental disorders, with their hundreds or thousands of interacting alleles.

Consider, for example, proposals for suicide prediction using data drawn from personal diaries in which patients report their thoughts (Melia et al., 2020). This idea is also naïve. Suicidal ideation is a very poor predictor of death by suicide. AI might do no better than the clinical measures that we already know to be limited in value. If we cannot reliably predict suicide with current tools, how can widening the database to include whether patients are thinking about or planning suicide reach this goal?

Thus, we face the same obstacles for therapy as we do for diagnosis. In principle, AI could be used to recommend evidence-based treatments. But as long as currently available options are not well understood, choices suggested by AI may not be better than what we already know – or don't know. While it AI could suggest changes in the molecules used in psychopharmacology, there is no guarantee they would work better than what we have now.

Finally, given the evidence that success in talking therapy depends on the personal skills of the psychotherapist (see Chapter 7), I am dubious about the future of AI as a provider of psychological treatment. While some trials found that sessions with a robot therapist can yield better outcomes than in wait-listed controls with little access to mental health care (Heinz et al., 2025), that is a very low bar.

A few years ago, I attended a reunion of medical classmates, and most of us agreed that the domain most likely to become dependent on AI would be radiology, and that the last one would be psychiatry. There may be a place for web-based advice about mental health, but we have had a large number of self-help books for decades without any reduction in the prevalence of psychopathology or the demand for treatment. (Just the opposite, I would think.)

The greatest opportunities for AI may lie in neuroscience. Its programs have the potential to make sense out of the enormous complexity of the brain connectome. If that could lead to valid predictions that have real clinical implications, then our long wait for a breakthrough might well be rewarded. I try to keep an open mind about this possibility, but suspect that only those who live into the 22nd century will see it happen. An even greater challenge for AI could be to provide more specific models of gene-environment interaction that are most likely to be the ultimate causes of psychopathology.

E.3 Are There Guides to the Future of Psychiatry?

The World Psychiatric Association (WPA) is a federation of national bodies in countries around the world. It publishes the most cited journal in our specialty, *World Psychiatry*. (It is also my favorite, as I prefer review articles and meta-analyses to single research reports that may or may not be replicated.)

Let us consider the findings of a WPA-Lancet Commission on the future of psychiatry, drawing on authors from all continents (Bhugra et al., 2017). This survey had much to say about access to care and discusses a number of issues that will affect psychiatric practice in the coming decades. One is that our patient population is changing, due to a shift to older, more urban, and migrant populations. Another is that psychiatry needs to find a better place in health care systems, using stepped care to distinguish between mild problems and severe disorders. Our specialty needs to move away from practice in private offices and to favor multidisciplinary teamwork. These changes are consistent with a public health approach that also supports the integration of mental and physical health care. Also recommended by this commission is that psychiatry needs an increased emphasis on social interventions and an engagement with wider societal issues, such as access to housing, resources, and employment. (Good luck with that!)

More realistically, services need access to good-quality care. Here digital technology might aid service delivery and the development of new treatments. Unfortunately, doing so could carry a risk for commercialized, unproven treatments. Finally, training in psychiatry demands programs in which new research is applied.

Some of these recommendations are commonsensical but require more than good intentions. Social interventions are certainly not what psychiatrists have been trained to do. They cost money and would only be available if society embraces and supports giving mental health a much higher priority.

How could we convince governments to adopt any of these ideas? For example, a pilot program across Canada offered better housing for patients with severe mental disorders, and the program was shown to be effective for better clinical stability (Aubry et al., 2016). But this hopeful initiative died once its initial funding expired.

It is not that psychiatrists fail to recognize problems in access to care. But our voices are not heard. That is where associations of the families of the mentally ill have more impact. This approach has been shown to work in the USA by National Alliance on Mental Illness (NAMI; Duckworth, 2022). If legislators knew more about psychiatry (perhaps from their own experience), then psychiatry would take a large step forward.

I conclude that a full acceptance of psychiatry and the reality of mental illness will remain an uphill battle. I have written this book with a focus on enduring challenges. Getting past these problems, as well as providing data that addresses unanswered questions, is not just around the corner. So we have to be patient. But I have little doubt that psychiatry will eventually make further progress – not soon but at some point over the next 50 years.

References

Abbass, A., Town, J., & Driessen, E. (2012). Intensive short-term dynamic psychotherapy: A systematic review and meta-analysis of outcome research. *Harvard Review of Psychiatry, 20*(2), 97–108.

Aceituno, D., Vera, N., Prina, A. M., & McCrone, P. (2019). Cost-effectiveness of early intervention in psychosis: Systematic review. *The British Journal of Psychiatry, 215*(1), 388–394.

Adamis, D., Flynn, C., Wrigley, M., Gavin, B., & McNicholas, F. (2022). ADHD in adults: A systematic review and meta-analysis of prevalence studies in outpatient psychiatric clinics. *Journal of Attention Disorders, 26*(12), 1523–1534.

Al-Dajani, N., Gralnick, T. M., & Bagby, R. M. (2016). A psychometric review of the Personality Inventory for DSM–5 (PID–5): Current status and future directions. *Journal of Personality Assessment, 98*(1), 62–81.

Altmann, U., Zimmermann, A., Kirchmann, H. A., Kramer, D., Fembacher, A., Bruckmayer, E., . . . & Strauss, B. M. (2016). Outpatient psychotherapy reduces healthcare costs: A study of 22,294 insurants over 5 years. *Frontiers in Psychiatry, 7*, 98.

Alwin, D. F. (2004). Parenting practices. In J. Scott, J. Treas, & M. Richards (Eds.), *The Blackwell companion to the sociology of families* (pp. 142–157). Malden, MA: Blackwell Publishing.

American Psychiatric Association. (1980). *Diagnostic and statistical manual of mental disorders (DSM-III)*. Washington, DC: American Psychiatric Press.

American Psychiatric Association. (2022). *Diagnostic and statistical manual of mental disorders, text revision (DSM-5-TR)*. Washington, DC: American Psychiatric Press.

Andersson, G., & Titov, N. (2014). Advantages and limitations of Internet-based interventions for common mental disorders. *World Psychiatry, 13*(1), 4–11.

Ang, M. J., Lee, S., Kim, J. C., Kim, S. H., & Moon, C. (2021). Behavioral tasks evaluating schizophrenia-like symptoms in animal models: A recent update. *Current Neuropharmacology, 19*(5), 641–664.

Angst, J. (1988). European long-term follow-up studies of schizophrenia. *Schizophrenia Bulletin, 14*(4), 501–513.

Appelbaum, P. S. (1992). Civil commitment from a systems perspective. *Law and Human Behavior, 16*(1), 61–74.

Appelbaum, P. S. (2017). Reflections on the Goldwater rule. *Journal of the American Academy of Psychiatry and the Law, 45*(2), 228–232.

Archer, J. (Ed.). (2022). *Male violence*. London: Taylor & Francis.

Aron, E. N., Aron, A., & Jagiellowicz, J. (2012). Sensory processing sensitivity: A review in the light of the evolution of biological responsivity. *Personality and Social Psychology Review, 16*(3), 262–282.

Arroll, B., Chin, W. Y., Martis, W., Goodyear-Smith, F., Mount, V., Kingsford, D., . . . & MacGillivray, S. (2016). Antidepressants for treatment of depression in primary care: A systematic review and meta-analysis. *Journal of Primary Health Care, 8*(4), 325–334.

Atkins Whitmer, D., & Woods, D. L. (2013). Analysis of the cost effectiveness of a suicide barrier on the Golden Gate Bridge. *Crisis, 34*(2), 98–106.

Aubry, T., Goering, P., Veldhuizen, S., Adair, C. E., Bourque, J., Distasio, J., . . . & Tsemberis, S. (2016). A multiple-city RCT of housing first with assertive community treatment for homeless Canadians with serious mental illness. *Psychiatric Services, 67*(3), 275–281.

Barbui, C., Purgato, M., Churchill, R., Adams, C., Amato, L., Macdonald, G., . . . & Sheriff,

R. S. (2017). Cochrane for global mental health. *The Lancet Psychiatry*, 4(4), e6.

Barlow, D. H., Harris, B. A., Eustis, E. H., & Farchione, T. J. (2020). The unified protocol for transdiagnostic treatment of emotional disorders. *World Psychiatry*, 19(2), 245.

Barsaglini, A., Sartori, G., Benetti, S., Pettersson-Yeo, W., & Mechelli, A. (2014). The effects of psychotherapy on brain function: A systematic and critical review. *Progress in Neurobiology*, 114, 1–14.

Batstra, L., & Frances, A. (2012). DSM-5 further inflates attention deficit hyperactivity disorder. *The Journal of Nervous and Mental Disease*, 200(6), 486–488.

Baumeister, R. F. (2002). Religion and psychology: Introduction to the special issue. *Psychological Inquiry*, 13(3), 165–167.

Baumeister, R. F. (2008). Free will in scientific psychology. *Perspectives on Psychological Science*, 3(1), 14–19.

Baumeister, R. F. (2024). *The science of free will: Bridging theory and positive psychology*. New York: Oxford University Press.

Baune, B. (Ed.). (2019). *Personalized psychiatry*. New York: Academic Press.

Baxter, A. J., Scott, K. M., Ferrari, A. J., Norman, R. E., Vos, T., & Whiteford, H. A. (2014). Challenging the myth of an "epidemic" of common mental disorders: Trends in the global prevalence of anxiety and hor between 1990 and 2010. *Depression and Anxiety*, 31(6), 506–516.

Beck, A. T., & Haigh, E. A. (2014). Advances in cognitive theory and therapy: The generic cognitive model. *Annual Review of Clinical Psychology*, 10(1), 1–24.

Belsky, J., Caspi, A., Moffitt, T. E., & Poulton, R. (2020). *The origins of you: How childhood shapes later life*. Cambridge, MA: Harvard University Press.

Belsky, J., & Pluess, M. (2009). Beyond diathesis stress: Differential susceptibility to environmental influences. *Psychological Bulletin*, 135(6), 885.

Bhugra, D., Tasman, A., Pathare, S., Priebe, S., Smith, S., Torous, J., . . . & Ventriglio, A. (2017). The WPA-Lancet Psychiatry Commission on the future of psychiatry. *The Lancet Psychiatry*, 4(10), 775–818.

Bishop, T. F., Press, M. J., Keyhani, S., & Pincus, H. A. (2014). Acceptance of insurance by psychiatrists and the implications for access to mental health care. *JAMA Psychiatry*, 71(2), 176–181.

Black, D. W. (2024). Update on antisocial personality disorder. *Current Psychiatry Reports*, 26(10), 543–549.

Blum, N., & Black, D. W. (2020). Systems Training for Emotional Predictability and Problem Solving (STEPPS) for the treatment of BPD. In N. Blum & D. W. Black, *Borderline personality disorder* (pp. 171–186). New York: Routledge.

Boesen, K., Paludan-Müller, A. S., Gøtzsche, P. C., & Jørgensen, K. J. (2022). Extended-release methylphenidate for attention deficit hyperactivity disorder (ADHD) in adults. *Cochrane Database of Systematic Reviews*, 2, CD012857.

Bolton, D. (2008). *What is mental disorder?: An essay in philosophy, science, and values*. New York: Oxford University Press.

Bolton, D. (2023). A revitalized biopsychosocial model: Core theory, research paradigms, and clinical implications. *Psychological Medicine*, 53(16), 7504–7511.

Bolton, D., & Gillett, G. (2019). *The biopsychosocial model of health and disease new philosophical and scientific developments*. Cham: Palgrave MacMillan.

Bommersbach, T. J., Johnson, G., Pazdernik, V. K., Bostwick, J. M., & McKean, A. J. (2025). Psychiatric prognosis following index suicide attempts in early adolescents. *JAMA Psychiatry*, 82(7), 728–733. DOI: 10 .1001/jamapsychiatry.2025.0673

Bommersbach, T. J., Olfson, M., & Rhee, T. G. (2024). National trends in emergency department visits for suicide attempts and intentional self-harm. *American Journal of Psychiatry*, 181(8), 741–752.

Bonabi, H., Müller, M., Ajdacic-Gross, V., Eisele, J., Rodgers, S., Seifritz, E., . . . & Rüsch, N. (2016). Mental health literacy, attitudes to help seeking, and perceived need as predictors of mental health service use: A longitudinal study. *The Journal of Nervous and Mental Disease, 204*(4), 321–324.

Bonanno, G. A. (2021). The resilience paradox. *European Journal of Psychotraumatology, 12*(1), 1942642.

Borsboom. (2017). A network theory of mental disorders. *World Psychiatry, 16,* 5–13.

Bower, P., & Gilbody, S. (2005). Stepped care in psychological therapies: Access, effectiveness and efficiency: Narrative literature review. *The British Journal of Psychiatry, 186*(1), 11–17.

Bozzatello, P., Blua, C., Brandellero, D., Baldassarri, L., Brasso, C., Rocca, P., & Bellino, S. (2024). Gender differences in borderline personality disorder: A narrative review. *Frontiers in Psychiatry, 15,* 1320546.

Breslau, J., Marshall, G. M., Pincus, H. A., & Brown, R. (2014). Are mental disorders more common in urban than rural areas of the United States? *Journal of Psychiatric Research, 56,* 50–55.

Brini, S., Brudasca, N. I., Hodkinson, A., Kaluzinska, K., Wach, A., Storman, D., ... & Bala, M. M. (2023). Efficacy and safety of transcranial magnetic stimulation for treating major depressive disorder: An umbrella review and re-analysis of published meta-analyses of randomised controlled trials. *Clinical Psychology Review, 100,* 102236.

Brouwers, M. C., Spithoff, K., Kerkvliet, K., Alonso-Coello, P., Burgers, J., Cluzeau, F., ... & Florez, I. D. (2020). Development and validation of a tool to assess the quality of clinical practice guideline recommendations. *JAMA Network Open, 3*(5), e205535.

Bulik, C. M., Coleman, J. R., Hardaway, J. A., Breithaupt, L., Watson, H. J., Bryant, C. D., & Breen, G. (2022). Genetics and neurobiology of eating disorders. *Nature Neuroscience, 25*(5), 543–554.

Button, K. S., Ioannidis, J. P., Mokrysz, C., Nosek, B. A., Flint, J., Robinson, E. S., & Munafò, M. R. (2013). Power failure: Why small sample size undermines the reliability

of neuroscience. *Nature Reviews Neuroscience, 14*(5), 365–376.

Bykov, K. V., Zrazhevskaya, I. A., Topka, E. O., Peshkin, V. N., Dobrovolsky, A. P., Isaev, R. N., & Orlov, A. M. (2022). Prevalence of burnout among psychiatrists: A systematic review and meta-analysis. *Journal of Affective Disorders, 308,* 47–64.

Byrne, D., & Callaghan, G. (2022). *Complexity theory and the social sciences: The state of the art.* New York: Routledge.

Cade, J. F. (1949). Lithium salts in the treatment of psychotic excitement. *Medical Journal of Australia, 2,* 349–352.

Cahalan, S. (2019). *The great pretender: The undercover mission that changed our understanding of madness.* New York, NY: Grand Central.

Calhoun, C. D., Stone, K. J., Cobb, A. R., Patterson, M. W., Danielson, C. K., & Bendezú, J. J. (2022). The role of social support in coping with psychological trauma: An integrated biopsychosocial model for posttraumatic stress recovery. *Psychiatric Quarterly, 93*(4), 949–970.

Campbell, A. (2013). *A mind of her own: The evolutionary psychology of women.* Oxford: Oxford University Press.

Carli, M., Kolachalam, S., Longoni, B., Pintaudi, A., Baldini, M., Aringhieri, S., ... & Scarselli, M. (2021). Atypical antipsychotics and metabolic syndrome: From molecular mechanisms to clinical differences. *Pharmaceuticals, 14*(3), 238.

Carlsson, A. (2001). A half-century of neurotransmitter research: Impact on neurology and psychiatry (Nobel lecture). *Chembiochem, 2*(7–8), 484–493.

Caspi, A., Houts, R. M., Belsky, D. W., Goldman-Mellor, S. J., Harrington, H., Israel, S., ... & Moffitt, T. E. (2014). The p factor: One general psychopathology factor in the structure of psychiatric disorders?. *Clinical Psychological Science, 2*(2), 119–137.

Caspi, A., McClay, J., Moffitt, T. E., Mill, J., Martin, J., Craig, I. W., ... & Poulton, R. (2002). Role of genotype in the cycle of violence in maltreated children. *Science, 297*(5582), 851–854.

Caspi, A., Sugden, K., Moffitt, T. E., Taylor, A., Craig, I. W., Harrington, H., . . . & Poulton, R. (2003). Influence of life stress on depression: Moderation by a polymorphism in the 5-HTT gene. *Science, 301*, 386–389.

Castaneda, A. E., Tuulio-Henriksson, A., Marttunen, M., Suvisaari, J., & Lönnqvist, J. (2008). A review on cognitive impairments in depressive and anxiety disorders with a focus on young adults, *Journal of Affective Disorders, 106*, 1–27.

Cervero, R. M., & Gaines, J. K. (2015). The impact of CME on physician performance and patient health outcomes: An updated synthesis of systematic reviews. *Journal of Continuing Education in the Health Professions, 35*(2), 131–138.

Chemtob, C. M., Hamada, R. S., Bauer, G., Kinney, B., & Torigoe, R. Y. (1988). Patients' suicides: Frequency and impact on psychiatrists. *The American Journal of Psychiatry, 145*(2), 224–228.

Chen, C. (2022). Recent advances in the study of the comorbidity of depressive and anxiety disorders. *Advances in Clinical and Experimental Medicine, 31*(4), 355–358.

Choi-Kain, L. W., Albert, E. B., & Gunderson, J. G. (2016). Evidence-based treatments for borderline personality disorder: Implementation, integration, and stepped care. *Harvard Review of Psychiatry, 24*, 342–356.

Cicchetti, D. (2023). A multiple levels of analysis developmental psychopathology perspective on adolescence and young adulthood. In L. J. Crockett, G. Carlo, & J. E. Schulenberg (Eds.), *APA handbook of adolescent and young adult development* (pp. 487–503). Washington, DC: American Psychological Association.

Cipriani, A., Furukawa, T. A., Salanti, G., Chaimani, A., Atkinson, L. Z., Ogawa, Y., . . . & Geddes, J. R. (2018). Comparative efficacy and acceptability of 21 antidepressant drugs for the acute treatment of adults with major depressive disorder: A systematic review and network meta-analysis. *The Lancet, 391*(10128), 1357–1366.

Cipriani, A., Hawton, K., Stockton, S., & Geddes, J. R. (2013). Lithium in the prevention of suicide in mood disorders: Updated systematic review and meta-analysis. *BMJ, 346*, f3646.

Cohen, Z. D., & DeRubeis, R. J. (2018). Treatment selection in depression. *Annual Review of Clinical Psychology, 14*(1), 209–236.

Connolly, K. R., & Thase, M. E. (2011). If at first you don't succeed: A review of the evidence for antidepressant augmentation, combination and switching strategies. *Drugs, 71*, 43–64.

Coombs, N. C., Meriwether, W. E., Caringi, J., & Newcomer, S. R. (2021). Barriers to healthcare access among U.S. adults with mental health challenges: A population-based study. *SSM, 15*, 100847.

Corrigan, P. W., Bink, A. B., Fokuo, J. K., & Schmidt, A. (2015). The public stigma of mental illness means a difference between you and me. *Psychiatry Research, 226*(1), 186–191.

Cortese, S., Kelly, C., Chabernaud, C., Proal, E., Di Martino, A., Milham, M. P., & Castellanos, F. X. (2012). Toward systems neuroscience of ADHD: A meta-analysis of 55 fMRI studies. *American Journal of Psychiatry, 169*(10), 1038–1055.

Cramer, V., Torgersen, S., & Kringlen, E. (2006). Personality disorders and quality of life. A population study. *Comprehensive Psychiatry, 47*(3), 178–184.

Cristea, I. A., Gentili, C., Cotet, C. D., Palomba, D., Barbui, C., & Cuijpers, P. (2017). Efficacy of psychotherapies for borderline personality disorder: A systematic review and meta-analysis. *JAMA Psychiatry, 74*(4), 319–328.

Cuijpers, P. (2024). How to improve outcomes of psychological treatment of depression: Lessons from "next-level" meta-analytic research. *American Psychologist, 79*(9), 1407.

Cuijpers, P., Harrer, M., Miguel, C., Ciharova, M., & Karyotaki, E. (2025). Five decades of research on psychological treatments of depression: A historical and meta-analytic overview. *American Psychologist, 80*(3), 297–310.

Cuijpers, P., Miguel, C., Harrer, M., Plessen, C. Y., Ciharova, M., Ebert, D., & Karyotaki, E.

(2023). Cognitive behavior therapy vs. control conditions, other psychotherapies, pharmacotherapies and combined treatment for depression: A comprehensive meta-analysis including 409 trials with 52,702 patients. *World Psychiatry, 22*(1), 105–115.

Cuijpers, P., Stringaris, A., & Wolpert, M. (2020). Treatment outcomes for depression: Challenges and opportunities. *The Lancet Psychiatry, 7*(11), 925–927.

Cumyn, L., French, L., & Hechtman, L. (2009). Comorbidity in adults with attention-deficit hyperactivity disorder. *The Canadian Journal of Psychiatry, 54*(10), 673–683.

Cunningham, J., & Shapiro, C. M. (2018): Cognitive Behavioural Therapy for Insomnia (CBT-I) to treat depression: A systematic review. *Journal of Psychosomatic Research, 106*, 1–12.

Cuthbert, B. N., & Insel, T. R. (2013). Toward the future of psychiatric diagnosis: The seven pillars of RDoC. *BMC Medicine, 11*, 1–8.

Dawkins, R. (1976): *The selfish gene.* Oxford: Oxford University Press.

De Crescenzo, F., D'Alò, G. L., Ostinelli, E. G., Ciabattini, M., Di Franco, V., Watanabe, N., . . . & Cipriani, A. (2022). Comparative effects of pharmacological interventions for the acute and long-term management of insomnia disorder in adults: A systematic review and network meta-analysis. *The Lancet, 400*(10347), 170–184.

De Moore, G. M., & Robertson, A. R. (1996). Suicide in the 18 years after deliberate self-harm: A prospective study. *British Journal of Psychiatry, 169*, 489–494.

De Rosa, C., Sampogna, G., Luciano, M., Del Vecchio, V., Fabrazzo, M., & Fiorillo, A. (2018). Social versus biological psychiatry: It's time for integration!. *International Journal of Social Psychiatry, 64*(7), 617–621.

Deak, J. D., & Johnson, E. C. (2021). Genetics of substance use disorders: A review. *Psychological Medicine, 51*(13), 2189–2200.

Dean, R. L., Hurducas, C., Hawton, K., Spyridi, S., Cowen, P. J., Hollingsworth, S., . . . & Cipriani, A. (2021): Ketamine and other glutamate receptor modulators for depression in adults with unipolar major depressive disorder. *Cochrane Database of Systematic Reviews,* (9), Article CD011612. DOI: 10.1002/14651858.CD011612.pub3

Del Giudice, M., & Haltigan, J. D. (2023). An integrative evolutionary framework for psychopathology. *Development and Psychopathology, 35*(1), 1–11.

Del Re, A. C., Spielmans, G. I., Flückiger, C., & Wampold, B. E. (2013). Efficacy of new generation antidepressants: Differences seem illusory. *PLoS One, 8*(6), e63509.

Dinicola, V. F. (1990). Anorexia multiforme: Self-starvation in historical and cultural context: Part II: Anorexia nervosa as a culture-reactive syndrome. *Transcultural Psychiatric Research Review, 27*(4), 245–286.

Docherty, J. R., & Alsufyani, H. A. (2021). Pharmacology of drugs used as stimulants. *The Journal of Clinical Pharmacology, 61,* S53–S69.

Dolnick, E. (1998). *Madness on the couch: Blaming the victim in the heyday of psychoanalysis.* New York: Simon and Schuster.

Duckworth, K. (2022). *You are not alone: The NAMI guide to navigating mental health— With advice from experts and wisdom from real people and families.* New York: Zando Publicatons.

Dunbar, R. I. (2009). The social brain hypothesis and its implications for social evolution. *Annals of Human Biology, 36*(5), 562–572.

Durkheim, E. (1979/1897). *Suicide: A study in sociology.* Trans. Spaulding, J. A. New York: The Free Press.

Eaton, N. R., Krueger, R. F., Keyes, K. M., Skodol, A. E., Markon, K. E., Grant, B. F., & Hasin, D. S. (2011). Borderline personality disorder co-morbidity: Relationship to the internalizing–externalizing structure of common mental disorders. *Psychological Medicine, 41*(5), 1041–1050.

Eaton, W. W., Martins, S. S., Nestadt, O. G., Bienvenu, J., Clarke, D., & Alexandre, P. (2008). *The burden of mental disorders. Epidemiologic Reviews, 30,* 1–14.

Engel, G. L. (1977). The need for a new medical model: A challenge for biomedicine. *Science, 196*(4286), 129–136.

Engel, L. G. (1980). The clinical application of the biopsychosocial model. *American Journal of Psychiatry, 137*(5), 535–544.

Erekson, D. M., Lambert, M. J., & Eggett, D. L. (2015). The relationship between session frequency and psychotherapy outcome in a naturalistic setting. *Journal of Consulting and Clinical Psychology, 83*(6), 1097–1107.

Fakra, E., & Azorin, J. M. (2012). Clozapine for the treatment of schizophrenia. *Expert Opinion on Pharmacotherapy, 13*(13), 1923–1935.

Farrell, M., Werge, T., & Sklar, P. (2015) Evaluating historical candidate genes for schizophrenia. *Molecular Psychiatry, 20*, 555–562.

Feldman, R., & Frondorf, E. (2017). *Drug wars: How big pharma raises prices and keeps generics off the market.* Cambridge: Cambridge University Press.

Fergusson, D. M., Boden, J. M., & Horwood, L. J. (2008). Exposure to childhood sexual and physical abuse and adjustment in early adulthood, *Child Abuse & Neglect, 32*, 607–619.

First, M. B., Bhat, V., Adler, D., Dixon, L., Goldman, B., Koh, S., … &. Siris, S. (2014). How do clinicians actually use the Diagnostic and Statistical Manual of Mental Disorders in clinical practice and why we need to know more. *The Journal of Nervous and Mental Disease, 202*, 841–844.

Fisher, H. L., Caspi, A., Moffitt, T. E., Wertz, J., Gray, R., Newbury, J., … & Arseneault, L. (2015). Measuring adolescents' exposure to victimization: The environmental risk (E-Risk) longitudinal twin study. *Development and Psychopathology, 27*(4pt2), 1399–1416.

Fitz-James, M. H., & Cavalli, G. (2022). Molecular mechanisms of transgenerational epigenetic inheritance. *Nature Reviews Genetics, 23*(6), 325–341.

Flint, J., & Kendler, K. S. (2014). The genetics of major depression. *Neuron, 81*, 484–503.

Fombonne, E. (2023). Is autism overdiagnosed? *Journal of Child Psychology and Psychiatry, 64*(5), 711–714.

Fornito, A., Bullmore, E. T., & Zalesky, A. (2017). Opportunities and challenges for psychiatry in the connectomic era. *Biological Psychiatry: Cognitive Neuroscience and Neuroimaging, 2*(1), 9–19.

Foucault, M., Murphy, J., & Khalfa, J. (2013). *History of madness.* New York: Routledge.

Fournier, J. C., DeRubeis, R. J., Hollon, S. D., Dimidjian, S., Amsterdam, J. D., Shelton, R. C., & Fawcett, J. (2010). Antidepressant drug effects and depression severity: A patient-level meta-analysis. *JAMA, 303*(1), 47–53.

Frances, A. (2013). *Saving normal.* New York: Morrow.

Frances, A. (2014). Resuscitating the biopsychosocial model. *The Lancet Psychiatry, 1*(7), 496–497.

Freud, S. (1937/1962). Analysis terminable and interminable: In J. Strachey, A. Freud, & C. L. Rothgeb (Eds.), *The standard edition of the psychological works of Sigmund Freud* (Vol. 23, pp. 216–254). London: Hogarth Pres.

Friedkin, N. E. (2004). Social cohesion. *Annual Review of. Sociology, 30*(1), 409–425.

Furedi, F. (2002). *Paranoid parenting: Why ignoring the experts may be best for your child.* Chicago: Chicago Review Press.

Furedi, F. (2017). *Therapeutic culture.* London: Routledge.

Galanter, M., & Kleber, H. D. (2011). *Psychotherapy for the treatment of substance abuse.* Washington, DC: American Psychiatric Publications.

Galvin, E., Desselle, S., Gavin, B., Quigley, E., Flear, M., Kilbride, K., … & Hayden, J. (2022). Patient and provider perspectives of the implementation of remote consultations for community-dwelling people with mental health conditions: A systematic mixed studies review, *Journal of Psychiatric Research, 156*, 668–678.

Gascon, A., Gamache, D., St-Laurent, D., & Stipanicic, A. (2022). Do we over-diagnose ADHD in North America? A critical review and clinical recommendations. *Journal of Clinical Psychology, 78*(12), 2363–2380.

Gaynes, B. N., Lux, L., Gartlehner, G., Asher, G., Forman-Hoffman, V., Green, J., ... & Lohr, K. N. (2020). Defining treatment-resistant depression. *Depression and Anxiety, 37*(2), 134–145.

GBD Collaborators, & Ärnlöv, J. (2020). Global burden of 87 risk factors in 204 countries and territories, 1990–2019: A systematic analysis for the Global Burden of Disease Study 2019. *The Lancet, 396*(10258), 1223–1249.

Geddes, J. R., Burgess, S., Hawton, K., Jamison, K., & Goodwin, G. M. (2004). Long-term lithium therapy for bipolar disorder: Systematic review and meta-analysis of randomized controlled trials. *American Journal of Psychiatry, 161*(2), 217–222.

Gerbasi, M. E., Richards, L. K., Thomas, J. J., Agnew-Blais, J. C., Thompson-Brenner, H., Gilman, S. E., & Becker, A. E. (2014). Globalization and eating disorder risk: Peer influence, perceived social norms, and adolescent disordered eating in Fiji. *International Journal of Eating Disorders, 47*(7), 727–737.

Germann, M., Brederoo, S. G., & Sommer, I. E. (2021). Abnormal synaptic pruning during adolescence underlying the development of psychotic disorders. *Current Opinion in Psychiatry, 34*(3), 222–227.

Ghaemi, S. N. (2011). The biopsychosocial model in psychiatry: A critique. *American Journal of Psychiatry, 121*(1), 451–457.

Giangrande, E. J., Weber, R. S., & Turkheimer, E. (2022). What do we know about the genetic architecture of psychopathology?. *Annual Review of Clinical Psychology, 18*(1), 19–42.

Gilbert, P. (1995). Biopsychosocial approaches and evolutionary theory as aids to integration in clinical psychology and psychotherapy. *Clinical Psychology & Psychotherapy, 2*(3), 135–156.

Gold, I. (2009). Reduction in psychiatry. *The Canadian Journal of Psychiatry, 54*(8), 506–512.

Goldbloom, D (2021): *We can do better: Urgent innovations to improve mental health access and care.* New York: Simon and Schuster.

Goodwin, F. K., & Jamison, K. R. (2007). *Manic-depressive illness: Bipolar disorders and recurrent depression* (2nd ed.). New York. Oxford University Press.

Gottesman, I. I., & Gould, T. D. (2003). The endophenotype concept in psychiatry: Etymology and strategic intentions. *American Journal of Psychiatry, 160*(4), 636–645.

Graber, J. A. (2013). Pubertal timing and the development of psychopathology in adolescence and beyond. *Hormones and Behavior, 64*(2), 262–269.

Grant, K. E., McMahon, S. D., Carter, J. S., Carleton, R. A., Adam, E. K., & Chen, E. (2014). The influence of stressors on the development of psychopathology. In M. Lewis & K. D. Rudolph (Eds.), *Handbook of developmental psychopathology* (pp. 205–223). Boston, MA: Springer US.

Gratzer, D., & Goldbloom, D. (2016). Making evidence-based psychotherapy more accessible in Canada. *The Canadian Journal of Psychiatry, 61*(10), 618–623.

Gratzer, D., & Khalid-Khan, F. (2016). Internet-delivered cognitive behavioural therapy in the treatment of psychiatric illness. *CMAJ, 188*(4), 263–272.

Gray, G. E. (2008). *Concise guide to evidence-based psychiatry.* Washington, DC: American Psychiatric Publishing.

Grenyer, B. F., Lewis, K. L., Fanaian, M., & Kotze, B. (2018). Treatment of personality disorder using a whole of service stepped care approach: A cluster randomized controlled trial. *PLoS One, 13*(11), e0206472.

Gross, J. J. (2015). Emotion regulation: Current status and future prospects. *Psychological Inquiry, 26*(1), 1–26.

Guerra-Farfan, E., Garcia-Sanchez, Y., Jornet-Gibert, M., Nuñez, J. H., Balaguer-Castro, M., & Madden, K. (2023). Clinical practice guidelines: The good, the bad, and the ugly. *Injury, 54,* S26–S29.

Gunderson, J. G., Stout, R. L., McGlashan, T. H., Shea, M. T., Morey, L. C., Grilo, C. M., ... & Skodol, A. E. (2011). Ten-year course of borderline personality disorder: Psychopathology and function from the

Collaborative Longitudinal Personality Disorders study. *Archives of General Psychiatry, 68*(8), 827–837.

Gupta, M. (2014). *Is evidence-based psychiatry ethical?* New York: Oxford University Press.

Gurland, B. J., Fleiss, J. L., Sharpe, L., Roberts, P., Cooper, J. E., & Kendell, R. E. (1970). Cross-national study of diagnosis of mental disorders: Hospital diagnoses and hospital patients in New York and London. *Comprehensive Psychiatry, 11*(1), 18–25.

Haidt, J. (2024). *The anxious generation.* New York: Penguin Press.

Haktanır, A., & Callender, K. A. (2020). Meta-analysis of dialectical behavior therapy (DBT) for treating substance use. *Research on Education and Psychology, 4*(Special Issue), 74–87.

Harris, J. R. (1998). *The nurture assumption: Why children turn out the way they do.* New York: Free Press.

Haslam, N. (2016). Concept creep: Psychology's expanding concepts of harm and pathology. *Psychological Inquiry, 27*(1), 1–17.

Havlik, J. L., Ososanya, L., Tang, D., Wahid, S., Ross, J. S., & Rhee, T. G. (2025). National trends in and concentration of industry payments to US Psychiatrists, 2015–2021. *Psychiatric Services, 76*(2), 210–213.

Hawton, K. (2014). Suicide prevention: A complex global challenge. *The Lancet Psychiatry, 1*(1), 2–3.

Healy, D. (2004). *The creation of psychopharmacology.* Cambridge, MA: Harvard University Press.

Hebb, D. O. (1949). *The organization of behavior: A neuropsychological theory.* New York: Wiley.

Heinz, M. V., Mackin, D. M., Trudeau, B. M., Bhattacharya, S., Wang, Y., Banta, H. A., . . . & Jacobson, N. C. (2025). Randomized trial of a generative AI Chatbot for mental health treatment. *NEJM AI, 2*(4), AIoa2400802.

Helle, A. C., Trull, T. J., Widiger, T. A., & Mullins-Sweatt, S. N. (2017). Utilizing interview and self-report assessment of the Five-Factor Model to examine convergence with the alternative model for personality disorders. *Personality Disorders: Theory, Research, and Treatment, 8*(3), 247.

Herpertz, S. C., Huprich, S. K., Bohus, M., Chanen, A., Goodman, M., Mehlum, L., . . . & Sharp, C. (2017). The challenge of transforming the diagnostic system of personality disorders. *Journal of Personality Disorders, 31*(5), 577–589.

Holliday, R. (2006). Epigenetics: A historical overview. *Epigenetics, 1*(2), 76–80.

Hollon, S. D. (2024). What we got wrong about depression and its treatment. *Behavior Research and Therapy, 180,* 104599.

Hollon, S. D., & Wampold, B. E. (2009). Are randomized controlled trials relevant to clinical practice? *The Canadian Journal of Psychiatry, 54*(9), 637–643.

Holst, Y., & Thorell, L. B. (2013). Neuropsychological functioning in adults with ADHD and adults with other psychiatric disorders: The issue of specificity. *Journal of Attention Disorders, 21*(2), 137–148.

Hopwood, C. J. (2019). Research and assessment with the AMPD. In C. J. Hopwood, A. L. Mulay, & M. H. Waugh (Eds.), *The DSM-5 alternative model for personality disorders* (pp. 77–95). New York: Routledge.

Horwitz, A. V., & Wakefield, J. (2007). *The loss of sadness: How psychiatry transformed normal sorrow into depressive disorder.* New York: Oxford University Press.

Horwitz, A. V., & Wakefield, J. (2012). *All we have to fear: Psychiatry's transformation of natural anxieties into mental disorder.* New York: Oxford University Press.

Howard, K. I., Kopta, S. M., Krause, M. S., & Orlinsky, D. E. (1986). The dose–effect relationship in psychotherapy. *American Psychologist, 41*(2), 159.

Hrdy, S. (2009). *Mothers and others: The evolutionary origins of mutual understanding.* Cambridge, MA: The Belknap Press of Harvard University Press

Hyde, J., Carr, H., Kelley, N., Seneviratne, R., Reed, C., Parlatini, V., . . . & Brandt, V. (2022). Efficacy of neurostimulation across mental disorders: Systematic review and meta-analysis of 208 randomized controlled trials. *Molecular Psychiatry, 27*(6), 2709–2719.

Hyman, S. E. (2021). Psychiatric disorders: Grounded in human biology but not natural kinds. *Perspectives in Biology and Medicine, 64*(1), 6–28.

Ingenhoven, T. J., & Duivenvoorden, H. J. (2011). Differential effectiveness of antipsychotics in borderline personality disorder: Meta-analyses of placebo-controlled, randomized clinical trials on symptomatic outcome domains. *Journal of Clinical Psychopharmacology, 31*(4), 489–496.

Insel, T. R. (2018). Digital phenotyping: A global tool for psychiatry. *World Psychiatry, 17*(3), 276.

Insel, T. R. (2022). *Healing: Our path from mental illness to mental health.* New York: Penguin Press.

Insel, T. R., & Cuthbert, B. N. (2015). "Brain disorders? Precisely." *Science, 348*(6234), 499–500.

Insel, T. R., & Quirion, R. (2005). Psychiatry as a clinical neuroscience discipline. *JAMA, 294*(17), 2221–2224.

Ioannidis, J. P. A. (2005). Why most published research findings are false. *PLoS Medicine, 2*(8), e124.

Ioannidis, J. P. A. (2012). Why science is not necessarily self-correcting. *Perspectives on Psychological Science, 7*(6), 645–654.

Ioannidis, J. P. A. (2017). Hijacked evidence-based medicine: Stay the course and throw the pirates overboard. *Journal of Clinical Epidemiology, 84*, 11–13.

Jang, K. L. (2005): *The behavioral genetics of psychopathology: A clinical guide.* New York: Routledge.

Jeitani, A., Fahey, P., Gascoigne, M., Darnal, A., & Lim, A. (2024): Effectiveness of stepped care for mental health disorders: An umbrella review of meta-analyses. *Personalized Medicine in Psychiatry, 47–48*, 100140.

Jericho, B., Luo, A., & Berle, D. (2022). Trauma-focused psychotherapies for post-traumatic stress disorder: A systematic review and network meta-analysis. *Acta Psychiatrica Scandinavica, 145*(2), 132–155.

Johnson, M., & Hyman, S. E. (2022). A critical perspective on the synaptic pruning hypothesis of schizophrenia pathogenesis. *Biological Psychiatry, 92*, 440–442.

Jones, P. B. (2013). Adult mental health disorders and their age at onset. *British Journal of Psychiatry, 202*(s54), s5–s10.

Jones, P. J., & McNally, R. J. (2022). Does broadening one's concept of trauma undermine resilience? *Psychological Trauma: Theory, Research, Practice, and Policy, 14*(S1), S131–S139.

Julien, C. (2015). Bourdieu, social capital and online interaction. *Sociology, 49*(2), 356–373.

Juul, S., Jakobsen, J. C., Jørgensen, C. K., Poulsen, S., Sørensen, P., & Simonsen, S. (2023). The difference between shorter- versus longer-term psychotherapy for adult mental health disorders: A systematic review with meta-analysis. *BMC Psychiatry, 23*(1), 438.

Kaess, M., Brunner, R., & Chaney, A. (2014). Borderline personality disorder in adolescence. *Pediatrics, 134*(4), 782–793.

Kagan, J. (1998). *Galen's prophecy: Temperament in human nature.* New York: Routledge.

Kahn, J. (2024). *Mastering AI: A survival guide to our superpowered future.* New York: Simon and Schuster.

Kazdin, A. E. (2018). *Innovations in psychosocial interventions and their delivery: Leveraging cutting-edge science to improve the world's mental health.* New York: Oxford University Press.

Keepers, G. A., Fochtmann, L. J., Anzia, J. M., Benjamin, S., Lyness, J. M., Mojtabai, R., . . . & Medicus, J. (2024). The American Psychiatric Association practice guideline for the treatment of patients with borderline personality disorder. *American Journal of Psychiatry, 181*(11), 1024–1028.

Kendler, K. S. (2005). Toward a philosophical structure for psychiatry. *American Journal of Psychiatry, 162*(3), 433–440.

Kendler, K. S. (2016). The nature of psychiatric disorders. *World Psychiatry, 15*(1), 5–12.

Kendler, K. S. (2019). From many to one to many: The search for causes of psychiatric illness. *JAMA Psychiatry, 76*(10), 1085–1091.

Kendler, K. S., & Gygnell, A. (2020). Multilevel interactions and the dappled causal world of psychiatric disorders. In W. Davies, J. Savulescu, R. Roache, & J. P. Loebell (Eds.), *Psychiatry reborn: Biopsychosocial psychiatry in modern medicine* (pp. 25–45). Oxford: Oxford University.

Kendler, K. S., Myers, J., & Zisook, S. (2008). Does bereavement-related major depression differ from major depression associated with other stressful life events? *American Journal of Psychiatry, 165*(11), 1449–1455.

Kendler, K. S., Ohlsson, H., Sundquist, K., & Sundquist, J. (2018). Sources of parent-offspring resemblance for major depression in a national Swedish extended adoption study. *JAMA Psychiatry, 75*(2), 194–200.

Kessler, R. C., Bossarte, R. M., Luedtke, A., Zaslavsky, A. M., & Zubizarreta, J. R. 2020. Suicide prediction models: A critical review of recent research with recommendations for the way forward. *Molecular Psychiatry, 25,* 168–179.

Kessler, R. C., McGonagle, K. A., Zhao, S., Nelson, C. B., Hughes, M., Eshleman, S., . . . & Kendler, K. S. (1994). Lifetime and 12-month prevalence of DSM-III-R psychiatric disorders in the United States: Results from the National Comorbidity Survey. *Archives of General Psychiatry, 51*(1), 8–19.

Khan, A., & Brown, W. A. (2015). Antidepressants versus placebo in major depression: An overview. *World Psychiatry, 14*(3), 294–300.

Killikelly, C., Smith, K. V., Zhou, B., Prigerson, H. G., O'Connor, M.-F., Kokou-Kpolou, C. K., . . . & Maercker, A. (2025). Prolonged grief disorder. *The Lancet.* DOI: 10.1016/S0140-6736(25)00354-X

Kingstone, E. (1960). The lithium treatment of hypomanic and manic states. *Comprehensive Psychiatry, 1,* 317–320.

Kirmayer, L. J., Lemelson, R., & Cummings, C. A. (Eds.). (2015). *Re-visioning psychiatry: Cultural phenomenology, critical neuroscience, and global mental health.* Cambridge: Cambridge University Press.

Kirsch, I. (2009). Antidepressants and the placebo response. *Epidemiology and Psychiatric Sciences, 18*(4), 318–322.

Kirsner, D. (2015). *The legacy of RD Laing.* New York: Routledge.

Kishi, T., Ikuta, T., Matsuda, Y., Sakuma, K., Okuya, M., Mishima, K., & Iwata, N. (2021). Mood stabilizers and/or antipsychotics for bipolar disorder in the maintenance phase: A systematic review and network meta-analysis of randomized controlled trials. *Molecular Psychiatry, 26*(8), 4146–4157.

Kivimaki, M., Batty, G. D., Penttti, J., & Shipley, M. J. (2020). Association between socioeconomic status and the development of mental and physical health conditions in adulthood: A multi-cohort study. *Lancet Public Health, 5,* e140–e149.

Krueger, R. F., Kotov, R., Watson, D., Forbes, M. K., Eaton, N. R., Ruggero, C. J., . . . & Zimmermann, J. (2018). Progress in achieving quantitative classification of psychopathology. *World Psychiatry, 17*(3), 282–293.

Kurdyak, P., Stukel, T. A., Goldbloom, D., Kopp, A., Zagorski, B. M., & Mulsant, B. H. (2014). Universal coverage without universal access: A study of psychiatrist supply and practice patterns in Ontario. *Open Medicine, 8*(3), e87.

Ladyman, J., Lambert, J., & Wiesner, K. (2013). What is a complex system? *European Journal of Philosophy of Science, 3,* 33–67.

Laporte, L., Paris, J., Zelkowitz, P., & Cardin, J. F. (2018). Clinical outcomes of a Stepped Care program for the treatment of borderline personality disorder. *Personality and Mental Health, 12,* 252–264.

Lasch, C. (1978). *The culture of narcissism.* New York. Norton.

Lazar, S. (Ed.). (2010). *Psychotherapy is worth it: A comprehensive review of its cost-effectiveness.* Washington, DC: American Psychiatric Publishing.

Legge, S. E., Santoro, M. L., Periyasamy, S., Okewole, A., Arsalan, A., Kowalec, K. (2021). Genetic architecture of schizophrenia: A review of major advancements. *Psychological Medicine*, *51*(13), 2168–2177.

Lehmann, H. E. (1958). Tranquillizers and other psychotropic drugs in clinical practice. *Canadian Medical Association Journal*, *79*(9), 701.

Lett, T. A., Vaidya, N., Jia, T., Polemiti, E., Banaschewski, T., Bokde, A. L. W., . . . & Schumann, G. (2025). Framework for brain-derived dimensions of psychopathology. *JAMA Psychiatry*, *82*(8), 778–789. DOI: 10.1001/jamapsychiatry.2025.1246

Leucht, S., Hierl, S., Kissling, W., Dold, M., & Davis, J. M. (2012). Putting the efficacy of psychiatric and general medicine medication into perspective: Review of meta-analyses. *The British Journal of Psychiatry*, *200*(2), 97–10.

Lieberman, J. A. (2015). *Shrinks: The untold story of psychiatry*. New York: Little, Brown and Company.

Lilienfeld, S. O., Ritschel, L. A., Lynn, S. J., Cautin, R. L., & Latzman, R. D. (2013). Why many clinical psychologists are resistant to evidence-based practice: Root causes and constructive remedies. *Clinical Psychology Review*, *33*, 883–900.

Linehan, M. M. (1993). *Cognitive behavior therapy for borderline personality disorder*. New York: Guilford.

Looi, J. C., Allison, S., Bastiampillai, T., Kisely, S., Maguire, P. A., Woon, L., & Anderson, K. (2025). Stopping antidepressants or not? *Australian Journal of General Practice*, *54*(3), 91–94.

Lumey, L. H. (2016). Long term health effects of the Dutch famine of 1944–1945: A summary of research findings. *The Royal Danish Academy of Sciences and Letters*, *4*(7), 115–124.

Lynall, M. E., & McIntosh, A. M. (2023). The heterogeneity of depression. *American Journal of Psychiatry*, *180*(10), 703–704.

Macey, D. (2019). *The lives of Michel Foucault*. Toronto: Verso Books.

Mackay, T. F., Stone, E. A., & Ayroles, J. F. (2009). The genetics of quantitative traits: Challenges and prospects. *Nature Reviews Genetics*, *10*(8), 565–577.

MacKillop, J., & Ray, L. A. (2017). The etiology of addiction: A contemporary biopsychosocial approach. In J. Mackillop & L. A. Ray (Eds.), *Integrating psychological and pharmacological treatments for addictive disorders* (pp. 32–53). New York: Routledge.

Mackinnon, S. P., Couture, M. E., Cooper, M. L., Kuntsche, E., O'Connor, R. M., Stewart, S. H., & DRINC Team. (2017). Cross-cultural comparisons of drinking motives in 10 countries: Data from the DRINC project. *Drug and Alcohol Review*, *36*(6), 721–730.

Malhi, G. S., Outhred, T., & Irwin, L. (2019): Bipolar II disorder is a myth. *The Canadian Journal of Psychiatry*, *64*(8), 531–536.

Marangoni, C., Hernandez, M., & Faedda, G. L. (2016). The role of environmental exposures as risk factors for bipolar disorder: A systematic review of longitudinal studies. *Journal of Affective Disorders*, *193*, 165–174.

Markham, M., Lutz, W., & Castonguay, L. (2021): *Bergin and Garfield's handbook of psychotherapy and behavior change*, 7th edition. New York: Wiley.

Markus, H. R., & Kitayama, S. (2003). Culture, self, and the reality of the social. *Psychological Inquiry*, *14*(3–4), 277–283.

Marrone, J., & Golowka, E. (1999). If work makes people with mental illness sick, what do unemployment, poverty, and social isolation cause? *Psychiatric Rehabilitation Journal*, *23*(2), 187–193.

Martínez-Alés, G., Jiang, T., Keyes, K. M., & Gradus, J. L. (2022). The recent rise of suicide mortality in the United States. *Annual Review of Public Health*, *43*(1), 99–116.

Maslej, M. M., Kloiber, S., Ghassemi, M., Yu, J., & Hill, S. L. (2023). Out with AI, in with the psychiatrist: A preference for human-derived clinical decision support in depression care. *Translational Psychiatry*, *13*(1), 210.

McGrath, J. J., Lim, C. C. W., Plana-Ripoll, O., Holtz, Y., Agerbo, E., Momen, N. C., … & de Jonge, P. (2020): Comorbidity within mental disorders: A comprehensive analysis based on 145 990 survey respondents from 27 countries. *Epidemiology and Psychiatric Sciences*, *12*(29), e153.

McHugh, P. R. (2008). *Try to remember: Psychiatry's clash over meaning, memory, and mind.* New York: Dana Press.

McLean, C. P., Levy, H. C., Miller, M. M., & Tolin, D. F. (2022): Exposure therapy for PTSD: A meta-analysis, *Clinical Psychology Review*, *91*, 102115.

McMain, S. F., Chapman, A. L., Kuo, J. R., Dixon-Gordon, K. L., Guimond, T. H., Labrish, C., … & Streiner, D. L. (2022). The effectiveness of 6 versus 12 months of dialectical behavior therapy for borderline personality disorder: A noninferiority randomized clinical trial. *Psychotherapy and Psychosomatics*, *91*(6), 382–397.

McNally, R. J. (2003). Progress and controversy in the study of posttraumatic stress disorder. *Annual Review of Psychology*, *54*(1), 229–252.

McNally, R. J. (2005). *Remembering trauma.* Cambridge, MA: Harvard University Press.

Meadows, G. N., Enticott, J. C., Inder, B., Russell, G. M., & Gurr, R. (2015). Better access to mental health care and the failure of the Medicare principle of universality. *Medical Journal of Australia*, *202*(4), 190–194.

Melia, R., Francis, K., Hickey, E., Bogue, J., Duggan, J., O'Sullivan, M., & Young, K. (2020). Mobile health technology interventions for suicide prevention: Systematic review. *JMIR mHealth and uHealth*, *8*(1), e12516.

Meltzer, H. Y., Alphs, L., Green, A. I., Altamura, A. C., Anand, R., Bertoldi, A., … & InterSePT Study Group. (2003). Clozapine treatment for suicidality in schizophrenia: International suicide prevention trial (InterSePT). *Archives of General Psychiatry*, *60*(1), 82–91.

Mercer, D., Douglass, A. B., & Links, P. S. (2009). Meta-analyses of mood stabilizers, antidepressants and antipsychotics in the treatment of borderline personality disorder: Effectiveness for depression and anger symptoms. *Journal of Personality Disorders*, *23*(2), 156–174.

Miresco, M. J., & Kirmayer, L. J. (2006). The persistence of mind-brain dualism in psychiatric reasoning about clinical scenarios. *American Journal of Psychiatry*, *163*(5), 913–918.

Mitchell, K. (2018). *Innate: How the wiring of our brains shapes who we are.* Princeton, NJ: Princeton University Press.

Mitchell, K. (2023). *Free agents: How evolution gave us free will.* Princeton, NJ: Princeton University Press.

Moffitt, T. E., Houts, R., Asherson, P., Belsky, D. W., Corcoran, D. L., Hammerle, M., …, & Caspi, A. (2015). Is adult ADHD a childhood-onset neurodevelopmental disorder? Evidence from a four-decade longitudinal cohort study. *American Journal of Psychiatry*, *172*(10), 967–977.

Moncrieff, J., Cooper, R. E., Stockmann, T., Amendola, S., Hengartner, M. P., & Horowitz, M. A. (2023). The serotonin theory of depression: A systematic umbrella review of the evidence. *Molecular Psychiatry*, *28*(8), 3243–3256.

Monteith, S., Glenn, T., Geddes, J., Whybrow, P. C., Achtyes, E., & Bauer, M. (2022). Expectations for artificial intelligence (AI) in psychiatry. *Current Psychiatry Reports*, *24*(11), 709–721.

Monteleone, A. M., & Abbate-Daga, G. (2024). Effectiveness and predictors of psychotherapy in eating disorders: State-of-the-art and future directions. *Current Opinion in Psychiatry*, *37*(6), 417–423.

Moreno-Agostino, D., Wu, T., Daskalopoulou, C., Hasan, T., Huisman, M., & Prina, M. (2021). Global trends in the prevalence and incidence of depression: A systematic review and meta-analysis. *Journal of Affective Disorders*, *281*, 235–243.

Moroz, N., Moroz, I., & D'Angelo, M. S. (2020). Mental health services in Canada: Barriers and cost-effective solutions to increase access. *Healthcare Management Forum*, *33*(6), 282–287.

Mottron, L. (2021). A radical change in our autism research strategy is needed: Back to prototypes. *Autism Research, 14*(10), 2213–2220.

Mueller, A. S., Abrutyn, S., Pescosolido, B., & Diefendorf, S. (2021). The social roots of suicide: Theorizing how the external social world matters to suicide and suicide prevention. *Frontiers in Psychology, 12,* 621569.

Mulder, R., & Tyrer, P. (2023). Borderline personality disorder: A spurious condition unsupported by science that should be abandoned. *Journal of the Royal Society of Medicine, 116*(4), 148–150.

Munafò, M. R., Durrant, C., Lewis, G., & Flint, J. (2009). Gene X environment interactions at the serotonin transporter locus. *Biological Psychiatry, 65*(3), 211.

Muttoni, S., Ardissino, M., & John, C. (2019). Classical psychedelics for the treatment of depression and anxiety: A systematic review. *Journal of Affective Disorders, 258,* 11–24.

Naghavi, M. (2019). Global, regional, and national burden of suicide mortality 1990 to 2016: Systematic analysis for the Global Burden of Disease Study 2016. *BMJ, 364,* 194.

National Center for Health Statistics. (2020). Antidepressant use among adults: United States, 2015–2018. https://www.cdc.gov/nchs/products/databriefs/db377.htm

National Institute for Clinical Excellence. (2018). 2018 Surveillance of personality disorders (NICE guidelines CG77 and CG78) surveillance report. www.nice.org

Nesse, R. M. (2023). Evolutionary psychiatry: Foundations, progress and challenges. *World Psychiatry, 22*(2), 177–202.

Newcomer, J. W., & Haupt, D. W. (2006). The metabolic effects of antipsychotic medication. *The Canadian Journal of Psychiatry, 51,* 480–491.

Njenga, C., Ramanuj, P. P., de Magalhães, F. J. C., & Pincus, H. A. (2024). New and emerging treatments for major depressive disorder. *BMJ, 386,* e073823.

Norcross, J. C., Beutler, L. E., & Levant, R. F. (2007). *Evidence-based practices in mental health.* Washington, DC: American Psychological Association.

Norcross, J. C., & Karpiak, C. P. (2024). Psychotherapy relationships. In S. Hupp & D. Tolin (Eds.), *Science-based therapy* (pp. 381–398). Cambridge: Cambridge University Press.

Norcross, J. C., & Lambert, M. J. (Eds.). (2019). *Psychotherapy relationships that work: Volume 1: Evidence-based therapist contributions* (pp. 381–398). Oxford: Oxford University Press.

Nordmo, M., Monsen, J. T., Høglend, P. A., & Solbakken, O. A. (2021). Investigating the dose–response effect in open-ended psychotherapy. *Psychotherapy Research, 31*(7), 859–869.

O'Donnell, M. (1997). *A sceptic's medical dictionary.* London: BMJ Publications.

Okolie, C., Wood, S., Hawton, K., Kandalama, U., Glendenning, A. C., Dennis, M., . . . & John, A. (2020): Means restriction for the prevention of suicide by jumping. *Cochrane Database of Systematic Reviews, 25*(2), CD013543.

Olfson, M., Blanco, C., Wang, S., & Greenhill, L. L. (2013). Trends in office-based treatment of adults with stimulants in the United States. *The Journal of Clinical Psychiatry, 74*(1), 21737.

Olfson, M., Gao, Y. N., Xie, M., Cullen, S. W., & Marcus, S. C. (2021). Suicide risk among adults with mental health emergency department visits with and without suicidal symptoms. *The Journal of Clinical Psychiatry, 82*(6), 37637.

Olfson, M., King, M., & Schoenbaum, M. (2015). Benzodiazepine use in the United States. *JAMA Psychiatry, 72*(2), 136–142.

Olfson, M., McClellan, C., Zuvekas, S. H., Wall, M., & Blanco, C. (2024). Trends in outpatient psychotherapy among adults in the US. *JAMA Psychiatry, 82*(3), 253–263.

Olfson, M., McClellan, C., Zuvekas, S. H., Wall, M., & Blanco, C. (2025). Psychotherapy trends in the United States. *American Journal of Psychiatry, 182*(5), 483–492.

O'Malley, S. S., Krishnan-Sarin, S., Farren, C., Sinha, R., & Kreek, M. (2002). Naltrexone decreases craving and alcohol self-administration in alcohol-dependent subjects and activates the hypothalamic–pituitary–adrenocortical axis. *Psychopharmacology, 160*, 19–29.

O'Nions, E., El Baou, C., & John, A. (2025): Life expectancy and years of life lost for adults with diagnosed ADHD in the UK: Matched cohort study. *The British Journal of Psychiatry, 226*, 1–8.

Ormel, J., Hollon, S. D., Kessler, R. C., Cuijpers, P., & Monroe, S. M. (2022). More treatment but no less depression: The treatment-prevalence paradox. *Clinical Psychology Review, 91*, 102111.

O'Sullivan, S. (2025). *The age of diagnosis: Sickness, health and why medicine has gone too far.* London: Hodder.

Pagura, J., Stein, M. B., Bolton, J. M., Cox, B. J., Grant, B., & Sareen, J. (2010). Comorbidity of borderline personality disorder and posttraumatic stress disorder in the U.S. population, *Journal of Psychiatric Research, 44*, 1190–1198.

Paris, J. (2009a). The bipolar spectrum: A critical perspective. *Harvard Review of Psychiatry, 17*(3), 206–213.

Paris, J. (2009b). The treatment of borderline personality disorder: Implications of research on diagnosis, etiology and outcome. *Annual Review of Clinical Psychology, 5*, 75–88.

Paris, J. (2012). *The bipolar spectrum.* New York: Routledge.

Paris, J. (2015a). *A concise guide to personality disorders.* Washington, DC: American Psychological Association Publishing.

Paris, J. (2015b). *The intelligent clinician's guide to the DSM-5.* Oxford: Oxford University Press.

Paris, J. (2017). *Stepped care for borderline personality disorder: Making treatment brief, effective, and accessible.* New York: Academic Press (Elsevier).

Paris, J. (2019). Dissociative identity disorder: Validity and use in the criminal justice system. *BJPsych Advances, 25*(5), 287–293.

Paris, J. (2020a). *Overdiagnosis in psychiatry: How modern psychiatry lost its way while creating a diagnosis for almost all of life's misfortunes.* Oxford: Oxford University Press.

Paris, J. (2020b). *Treatment of borderline personality disorder: A guide to evidence-based practice, 2nd edition, revised and updated,* New York: Guilford Press.

Paris, J. (2020c). *Social factors in personality disorders,* 2nd edition. Cambridge: Cambridge University Press.

Paris, J. (2022a). *Fad and fallacies in psychiatry,* 2nd edition. Cambridge, UK: Cambridge University Press.

Paris, J. (2022b). *Nature and nurture in personality and psychopathology: A guide for clinicians.* New York: Routledge.

Paris, J. (2022c). *Myths of trauma.* New York: Oxford University Press.

Paris, J. (2022d). Why electroconvulsive therapy still carries a stigma. Commentary on "Shock tactics, ethics, and fear: An academic and personal perspective on the case against ECT." *The British Journal of Psychiatry, 3*, 113–114.

Paris, J. (2023a). Personality. In S. Hupp, & C. Cara Santa Maria (Eds.), *Pseudoscience in therapy: A skeptical field guide* (pp. 247–260). Cambridge: Cambridge University Press.

Paris, J. (2023b). *Half in love with death,* 2nd edition. New York: Routledge.

Paris, J. (2023c). Complex post-traumatic stress disorder and a biopsychosocial model of borderline personality disorder. *Journal of Nervous and Mental Disease, 211,* 805–810.

Paris, J. (2024). *Prescriptions for the mind,* 2nd edition. New York: Oxford University Press.

Paris, J. (2025). *A concise guide to borderline personality disorder.* Washington, DC: American Psychological Association Publishing.

Paris, J., Bhat, V., & Thombs, B. (2015a). Is adult attention-deficit hyperactivity disorder being overdiagnosed?. *Canadian Journal of Psychiatry, 60*(7), 324–328.

Paris, J., Goldbloom, D., & Kurdyak, P. (2015b). Moving out of the office:

Removing barriers to access to psychiatrists. *The Canadian Journal of Psychiatry*, 60(9), 403–406.

Paris, J., & Kirmayer, L. J. (2016). The National Institute of Mental Health research domain criteria: A bridge too far. *The Journal of Nervous and Mental Disease*, 204(1), 26–32.

Paris, J., & Zweig-Frank, H. (2001). A 27 year follow-up of patients with borderline personality disorder. *Comprehensive Psychiatry*, 42, 482–487.

Parker, G. (2000). Classifying depression: Should paradigms lost be regained?. *American Journal of Psychiatry*, 157(8), 1195–1203.

Parker, G. (2005). Beyond major depression. *Psychological Medicine*, 35(4), 467–474.

Parnas, J. (2014). The RDoC program: Psychiatry without psyche? *World Psychiatry*, 13(1), 46.

Perera, T., George, M. S., Grammer, G., Janicak, P., Pascual-Leone, A., & Wirecki, T. S. (2016). The Clinical TMS Society consensus review and treatment recommendations for TMS therapy for major depressive disorder. *Brain Stimulation*, 9, 336–346.

Pigoni, A., Delvecchio, G., Turtulici, N., Madonna, D., Pietrini, P., Cecchetti, L., & Brambilla, P. (2024). Machine learning and the prediction of suicide in psychiatric populations: A systematic review. *Translational Psychiatry*, 14(1), 140.

Pincus, H. A., Tew, Jr., J. D., & First, M. B. (2004). Psychiatric comorbidity: Is more less? *World Psychiatry*, 3(1), 18.

Pine, D. S., & Fox, N. A. (2015). Childhood antecedents and risk for adult mental disorders. *Annual Review of Psychology*, 66(1), 459–485.

Pinker, S. (2002). *The blank slate: The modern denial of human nature*. New York: Putnam Penguin.

Pinker, S. (2011). *The better angels of our nature: The decline of violence in history and its causes*. London: Penguin.

Plackett, R., Sheringham, J., & Dykxhoorn, J. (2023). The longitudinal impact of social media use on UK adolescents' mental health: Longitudinal observational study. *Journal of Medical Internet Research*, 25, e43213.

Plomin, R., Gidziela, A., Malanchini, M., & Von Stumm, S. (2022). Gene–environment interaction using polygenic scores: Do polygenic scores for psychopathology moderate predictions from environmental risk to behavior problems?. *Development and Psychopathology*, 34(5), 1816–1826.

Poulton, R., Guiney, H., Ramrakha, S., & Moffitt, T. E. (2023). The Dunedin study after half a century: Reflections on the past, and course for the future. *Journal of the Royal Society of New Zealand*, 53(4), 446–465.

Powell, J., Geddes, J., Deeks, J., Goldacre, M., & Hawton, K. (2000). Suicide in psychiatric hospital in-patients: Risk factors and their predictive power. *British Journal of Psychiatry*, 176(3), 266–272.

Presskreischer, R., Barry, C. L., Lawrence, A. K., McCourt, A., Mojtabai, R., & McGinty, E. E. (2023). Factors affecting state-level enforcement of the Federal Mental Health Parity and Addiction Equity Act: A cross-case analysis of four states. *Journal of Health Politics, Policy and Law*, 48(1), 1–34.

Rapoport, J. L., Buchsbaum, M. S., Zahn, T. P., Weingartner, H., Ludlow, C., & Mikkelsen, E. J. (1978). Dextroamphetamine: Cognitive and behavioral effects in normal prepubertal boys. *Science*, 199, 560–563.

Redding, R. E. (2023). Psychologists' politics. In: C. L. Frisby, R. E. Redding, W. T. O'Donohue, & S. O. Lilienfeld (Eds.), *Ideological and political bias in psychology* (pp. 1–14). New York: Springer.

Regier, D. A., Narrow, W. E., Clarke, D. E., Kraemer, H. C., Kuramoto, S. J., Kuhl, E. A., & Kupfer, D. J. (2013). DSM-5 field trials in the United States and Canada, Part II: Test-retest reliability of selected categorical diagnoses. *American Journal of Psychiatry*, 170(1), 59–70.

Reinert, M., Fritze, D., & Nguyen, T. (2024). The state of mental health in America 2024. Alexandria VA: Mental Health America.

Rende, R., & Plomin, R. (1992). Diathesis-stress models of psychopathology:

A quantitative genetic perspective. *Applied and Preventive Psychology, 1*(4), 177–182.

Ribeiro, J. P., Juul, S., Kongerslev, M. T., Jørgensen, M. S., Völlm, B. A., Edemann-Callesen, H., … & Storebø, O. J. (2024). Pharmacological interventions for co-occurring psychopathology in people with borderline personality disorder: Secondary analysis of the Cochrane systematic review with meta-analyses. *The British Journal of Psychiatry, 226*(4), 226–237.

Ribeiro, W. S., Bauer, A., Andrade, M., York-Smioth, M., Pan, P. M., Pingani, L., … & Evans-Lacko, S. (2017). Income inequality and mental illness-related morbidity and resilience: A systematic review and meta-analysis *Lancet Psychiatry, 4*, 554–562.

Ritchie, S. (2020). *Science fictions.* New York: Henry Holt.

Roberts, B. W., Luo, J., Briley, D. A., Chow, P. I., Su, R., & Hill, P. L. (2017). A systematic review of personality trait change through intervention. *Psychological Bulletin, 143*(2), 117.

Rogers, C. R. (1995). *On becoming a person: A therapist's view of psychotherapy.* Boston: Houghton Mifflin Harcourt.

Romans, S. E., & Seeman, M. V. (Eds.). (2006). *Women's mental health: A life-cycle approach.* Baltimore: Lippincott Williams & Wilkins.

Rosenhan, D. L. (1973). On being sane in insane places. *Science, 179*(4070), 250–258.

Rosenzweig, E. (2016). With eyes wide open: How and why awareness of the psychological immune system is compatible with its efficacy. *Perspectives on Psychological Science, 11*(2), 222–238.

Ross, L. (2018). From the fundamental attribution error to the truly fundamental attribution error and beyond: My research journey. *Perspectives on Psychological Science, 13*(6), 750–769.

Rowland, A. S., Skipper, B. J., Umbach, D. M., Rabiner, D. L., Campbell, R. A., Naftel, A. J., & Sandler, D. P. (2013). The Prevalence of ADHD in a Population-Based Sample. *Journal of Attention Disorders, 19*(9), 741–754.

Rowland, T. A., & Marwaha, S. (2018). Epidemiology and risk factors for bipolar disorder. *Therapeutic Advances in Psychopharmacology, 8*(9), 251–269.

Rüsch, N. (2022). *The stigma of mental illness: Strategies against social exclusion and discrimination.* London: Elsevier.

Rush, A. J. (2023). Challenges of research on treatment-resistant depression: A clinician's perspective. *World Psychiatry, 22*(3), 415.

Rust, N. C. (2025). *Elusive cures: Why neuroscience hasn't solved brain disorders—And how we can change that.* New York: Henry Holt.

Rutter, M. (2005). How the environment affects mental health. *The British Journal of Psychiatry, 186*(1), 4–6.

Rutter, M. (2006). *Genes and behavior: Nature-nurture interplay explained.* London, UK: Blackwell.

Rutter, M. (2013). Annual research review: Resilience–clinical implications. *Journal of Child Psychology and Psychiatry, 54*(4), 474–487.

Rutter, M., Beckett, C., Castle, J., Colvert, E., Kreppner, J., Mehta, M., … & Sonuga-Barke, E. (2007). Effects of profound early institutional deprivation: An overview of findings from a UK longitudinal study of Romanian adoptees. *European Journal of Developmental Psychology, 4*(3), 332–350.

Rybakowski, J. K. (2020). Lithium–past, present, future. *International Journal of Psychiatry in Clinical Practice, 24*(4), 330–340.

Sackett, D. L., Rosenberg, W. M., Gray, J. M., Haynes, R. B., & Richardson, W. S. (1996). Evidence based medicine: What it is and what it isn't. *BMJ, 312*(7023), 71–72.

Sandford, D. M., Kirtley, O. J., Thwaites, R., & O'Connor, R. C. (2021). The impact on mental health practitioners of the death of a patient by suicide: A systematic review. *Clinical Psychology & Psychotherapy, 28*(2), 261–294.

Santhouse, A. (2025). *No more normal: Mental health in an age of over-diagnosis.* London: Granta.

Satel, S., & Lilienfeld, S. O. (2013). *Brainwashed: The seductive appeal of mindless neuroscience*. Cambridge: Basic Civitas Books.

Savulescu, J., Roache, R., Davies, W., & Loebel, J. P. (Eds.). (2020). *Psychiatry reborn: Biopsychosocial psychiatry in modern medicine*. New York: Oxford University Press.

Sawaya, H., Miller, J. C., & Raines, J. M. (2024). Review of studies on incremental validity of assessment measures used in psychological assessment of attention-deficit hyperactivity disorder. *Assessment, 31*(2), 518–537.

Scheff, T. J. (2017). *Being mentally ill: A sociological study*. New York: Routledge.

Scheiderer, E. M., Wood, P. K., & Trull, T. J. (2015). The comorbidity of borderline personality disorder and posttraumatic stress disorder: Revisiting the prevalence and associations in a general population sample. *Borderline Personality Disorder and Emotion Dysregulation, 2*, 1–16.

Schou, M., Juel-Nielsen, N., Strömgren, E., & Voldby, H. (1954). The treatment of manic psychoses by the administration of lithium salts. *Journal of Neurology, Neurosurgery, and Psychiatry, 17*(4), 250.

Scott, K. M., Koenen, K. C., King, A., Petukhova, M. V., Alonso, J., Bromet, E. J., Bruffaerts, R., . . . & Kessler, R. C. (2018). Post-traumatic stress disorder associated with sexual assault among women in the WHO World Mental Health Surveys. *Psychological Medicine, 48*(1), 155–167.

Scott, M. J. (2025). 'Thanks, but no thanks': The public's response to engagement with NHS Talking Therapies–A salutary tale? *Counselling and Psychotherapy Research, 25*, e12852.

Scull, A. (2023). Rosenhan revisited: Successful scientific fraud. *History of Psychiatry, 34*(2), 180–195.

Seiden, R. H. (1978). Where are they now? A follow-up study of suicide attempters from the Golden Gate Bridge. *Suicide and Life-Threatening Behavior, 8*(4), 203–216.

Selten, J. P., & Cantor-Graae, E. (2007). Hypothesis: Social defeat is a risk factor for schizophrenia? *The British Journal of Psychiatry, 191*(S51), s9–s12.

Selten, J. P., van der Ven, E., & Termorshuizen, F. (2020). Migration and psychosis: A meta-analysis of incidence studies. *Psychological Medicine, 50*(2), 303–313.

Shekouh, D., Sadat Kaboli, H., Ghaffarzadeh-Esfahani, M., Khayamdar, M., Hamedani, Z., Oraee-Yazdani, S., . . . & Amanzadeh, E. (2024). Artificial intelligence role in advancement of human brain connectome studies. *Frontiers in Neuroinformatics, 18*, 1399931.

Shorter, E. (1992). *From paralysis to fatigue*. New York: Wiley.

Sibley, M. H., Arnold, L. E., Swanson, J. M., Hechtman, L. T., Kennedy, T. M., Owens, E., . . . & MTA Cooperative Group. (2022). Variable patterns of remission from ADHD in the multimodal treatment study of ADHD. *American Journal of Psychiatry, 179*(2), 142–151.

Silverman, J. L., Thurm, A., Ethridge, S. B., Soller, M. M., Petkova, S. P., Abel, T., . . . & Halladay, A. (2022). Reconsidering animal models used to study autism spectrum disorder: Current state and optimizing future. *Genes, Brain and Behavior, 21*(5), e12803.

Simonsen, E., & Paris, J. (2025). The borderline specifier. In B. Bach (Ed.), *ICD-11 personality disorders; assessment and treatment* (pp. 69–84). New York: Oxford University Press.

Sinyor, M., Men, V. Y., Chan, P. P. M., Sanchez Morales, D., Levitt, A. J., & Schaffer, A. (2024). Long-term impact of the Bloor Viaduct Suicide Barrier on suicides in Toronto: A time-series analysis. *The Canadian Journal of Psychiatry, 70*(4), 328–334.

Smit, Y., Huibers, M., Ioannididis, J., van Dyck, R., van Tilburg, W., & Arntz, A. (2012). The effectiveness of long-term psychoanalytic psychotherapy: A meta-analysis of randomized controlled trials. *Clinical Psychology Review, 32*, 81–92.

Smith, M. L., Glass, G. V., & Miller, T. (1980). *The benefits of psychotherapy*. Baltimore: Johns Hopkins Press.

Smith, O. R., Clark, D. M., Hensing, G., Layard, R., & Knapstad, M. (2025). Cost-benefit of IAPT Norway and effects on work-related outcomes and health care utilization: Results from a randomized controlled trial using registry-based data. *Psychological Medicine, 55,* e86.

Smith-Apeldoorn, S. Y., Veraart, J. K. E., Spijker, J., Kamphuis, J., & Schoevers, R. A. (2022). Maintenance ketamine treatment for depression: A systematic review of efficacy, safety, and tolerability. *The Lancet Psychiatry, 9*(11), 907–921.

Smolak, L., & Levine, M. P. (2015). Toward an integrated biopsychosocial model of eating disorders. In L. Smolak & M. P. Levine (Eds.), *The Wiley handbook of eating disorders* (pp. 929–941). New York: Wiley.

Smoller, J. W. (2017). A quarter century of progress in psychiatric genetics. *Harvard Review of Psychiatry, 25*(6), 256–258.

Smoller, J. W., Andreassen, O. A., Edenberg, H. J., Faraone, S. V., Glatt, S. J., & Kendler, K. S. (2019). Psychiatric genetics and the structure of psychopathology. *Molecular Psychiatry, 24*(3), 409–420.

Spock, B. (1946). *The common sense book of baby and child care.* New York: Duell, Sloan & Pearce.

Spoelma, M. J., Serafimovska, A., & Parker, G. (2023). Differentiating melancholic and non-melancholic depression via biological markers: A review. *The World Journal of Biological Psychiatry, 24*(9), 761–810.

Spring, B. (2007). Evidence-based practice in clinical psychology: What it is, why it matters; what you need to know. *Journal of Clinical Psychology, 63*(7), 611–631.

Srole, L., & Fischer, A. K. (2021). Gender, generations, and well-being: The Midtown Manhattan longitudinal study. In L. Erlenmeyer-Kimling & N. E. Miller (Eds.), *Life-span research on the prediction of psychopathology* (pp. 223–237). New York: Routledge.

Stein, D. J., Shoptaw, S. J., Vigo, D. V., Lund, C., Cuijpers, P., Bantjes, J., … & Maj, M. (2022). Psychiatric diagnosis and treatment in the Twenty-first century: Paradigm shifts versus incremental integration. *World Psychiatry, 21*(3), 393–414.

Stein, M. B., Jang, K. L., Taylor, S., Vernon, P. A., & Livesley, W. J. (2002). Genetic and environmental influences on trauma exposure and posttraumatic stress disorder symptoms: A twin study. *American Journal of Psychiatry, 159*(10), 1675–1681.

Stern, A. (1938). Psychoanalytic investigation of and therapy in the borderline Group of Neuroses. *Psychoanalytic Quarterly, 7*(4), 467–489.

Stoffers-Winterling, J., Storebø, O. J., & Lieb, K. (2020). Pharmacotherapy for borderline personality disorder: An update of published, unpublished and ongoing studies. *Current Psychiatry Reports, 22,* 1–10.

Storebø, O. J., Stoffers-Winterling, J. M., Völlm, B. A., Kongerslev, M. T., Mattivi, J. T., Kielsholm, M. L., … & Simonsen E. (2018): Psychological therapies for people with borderline personality disorder. *Cochrane Database of Systematic Reviews,* (2), CD012955. DOI: 10.1002/14651858. CD012955

Strickhouser, J. E., Zell, E., & Krizan, Z. (2017). Does personality predict health and well-being? A metasynthesis. *Health Psychology, 36*(8), 797–810.

Strupp, H. H., Fox, R. E., & Lesser, K. (1969). *Patients view their psychotherapy.* Baltimore: Johns Hopkins Press.

Su, Y., Li, M., Caron, J., Li, D., & Meng, X. (2024). Differential effects of lifetime stressors on major depressive disorder severity: A longitudinal community-based cohort study. *European Psychiatry, 67*(1), e66.

Suokas, J., Suominen, K., Isometsa, E., Ostamo, A., & LoÈnnqvist, J. (2001). Long-term risk factors for suicide mortality after attempted suicide: Findings of a 14-year follow-up study. *Acta Psychiatrica Scandinavica, 104,* 117–121.

Swanepoel, A. (2024). ADHD and ASD are normal biological variations as part of human evolution and are not "disorders." *Clinical Neuropsychiatry, 21*(6), 451.

Szasz, T. S. (1960). The myth of mental illness. *American Psychologist, 15*(2), 113.

Tacoli, C., McGranahan, G., & Satterthwaite, D. (2015). *Urbanisation, rural-urban migration and urban poverty* (Vol. 1). London: Human Settlements Group, International Institute for Environment and Development.

Taleb, N. N. (2007). *The black swan: The impact of the highly improbable.* New York: Random House.

Taylor, M. A. (2013). *Hippocrates cried: The decline of American psychiatry.* New York: Oxford University Press.

Tidemalm, D., Långström, N., Lichtenstein, P., & Runeson, B. (2008). Risk of suicide after suicide attempt according to coexisting psychiatric disorder: Swedish cohort study with long term follow-up. *BMJ, 337*, a2205.

Trifu, S., Sevcenco, A., Stănescu, M., Drăgoi, A. M., & Cristea, M. B. (2021). Efficacy of electroconvulsive therapy as a potential first-choice treatment in treatment-resistant depression. *Experimental and Therapeutic Medicine, 22*(5), 1281.

True, W. R., Rice, J., Eisen, S. A., Heath, A. C., Goldberg, J., Lyons, M. J., & Nowak, J. (1993). A twin study of genetic and environmental contributions to liability for posttraumatic stress symptoms. *Archives of General Psychiatry, 50*(4), 257–264.

Truijens, F., Zühlke-van Hulzen, L., & Vanheule, S. (2019). To manualize, or not to manualize: Is that still the question? A systematic review of empirical evidence for manual superiority in psychological treatment. *Journal of Clinical Psychology, 75*(3), 329–343.

Trull, T. J., Jahng, S., Tomko, R. L., Wood, P. K., & Sher, K. J. (2010). Revised NESARC personality disorder diagnoses: Gender, prevalence, and comorbidity with substance dependence disorders. *Journal of Personality Disorders, 24*(4), 412–426.

Turecki, G., Brent, D. A., Gunnell, D., O'Connor, R. C., Oquendo, M. A., Pirkis, J., & Stanley, B. H. (2019). Suicide and suicide risk. *Nature Reviews Disease Primers, 5*(1), 74.

Turkheimer, E. (2000). Three laws of behavior genetics and what they mean. *Current Directions in Psychological Science, 9*(5), 160–164.

Turkheimer, E. (2024). *Understanding the nature-nurture debate.* Cambridge: Cambridge University Press.

Turkheimer, E., Pettersson, E., & Horn, E. E. (2014). A phenotypic null hypothesis for the genetics of personality. *Annual Review of Psychology, 65*(1), 515–540.

Turner, B. O., Paul, E. J., Miller, M. B., & Barbey, A. K. (2018). Small sample sizes reduce the replicability of task-based fMRI studies. *Communications Biology, 1*, 62.

Turner, R. J., & Turner, J. B. (1999). Social integration and support. In C. S. Aneshensel, J. C. Phelan, & A. Bierman (Eds.), *Handbook of the sociology of mental health* (pp. 301–309). Boston, MA: Springer.

Twenge, J. M. (2023). *Generations: The real differences between Gen Z, Millennials, Gen X, Boomers, and Silents – And what they mean for America's future.* New York: Simon and Schuster.

Tyrer, P. (2014). Borderline personality disorder and mood. *The British Journal of Psychiatry, 205*(2), 161–162.

Van, H. L., & Kool, M. (2018). What we do, do not, and need to know about comorbid depression and personality disorders. *The Lancet Psychiatry, 5*(10), 776–778.

Van der Kolk, B. (2015). *The body keeps the score: brain, mind, and body in the healing of trauma.* New York: Penguin.

van Straten, A., Hill, J., Richards, D. A., & Cuijpers, P. (2015). Stepped care treatment delivery for depression: A systematic review and meta-analysis. *Psychological Medicine, 45*(2), 231–246.

Varin, M., Orpana, H. M., Palladino, E., Pollock, N. J., & Baker, M. M. (2021). Trends in suicide mortality in Canada by sex and age group, 1981 to 2017: A population-based time series analysis. *The Canadian Journal of Psychiatry, 66*(2), 170–178.

Villas Boas, P. J., Spagnuolo, R. S., Kamegasawa, A., Braz, L. G., do Valle, A. P., Jorge, E. C., ... & El Dib, R. (2013).

Systematic reviews showed insufficient evidence for clinical practice in 2004: What about in 2011? The next appeal for the evidence-based medicine age. *Journal of Evaluation in Clinical Practice, 19*(4), 633–637.

Wade, D. T., & Halligan, P. W. (2017). The biopsychosocial model of illness: A model whose time has come. *Clinical Rehabilitation, 31*(8), 995–1004.

Wakefield, J. C. (2007). The concept of mental disorder: Diagnostic implications of the harmful dysfunction analysis. *World Psychiatry, 6*(3), 149.

Wakefield, J. C. (2013). The DSM-5 debate over the bereavement exclusion: Psychiatric diagnosis and the future of empirically supported treatment. *Clinical Psychology Review, 33*(7), 825–845.

Walsh, C. G., Ribeiro, J. D., & Franklin, J. C. (2017). Predicting risk of suicide attempts over time through machine learning. *Clinical Psychological Science, 5*(3), 457–469.

Wampold, B. E., & Imel, Z. E. (2015). *The great psychotherapy debate: The evidence for what makes psychotherapy work.* New York: Taylor and Francis.

Wang, B., Feldman, I., Chkonia, E., Pinchuk, I., Panteleeva, L., & Skokauskas, N. (2022). Mental health services in Scandinavia and Eurasia: Comparison of financing and provision. *International Review of Psychiatry, 34*(2), 118–127.

Wazana, A. (2000). Physicians and the pharmaceutical industry: Is a gift ever just a gift?. *JAMA, 283*(3), 373–380.

Wertz, J., Caspi, A., Belsky, D. W., Beckley, A. L., Arseneault, L., Barnes, J. C., . . . & Moffitt, T. E. (2018). Genetics and crime: Integrating new genomic discoveries into psychological research about antisocial behavior. *Psychological Science, 29*(5), 791–803.

Westen, D., & Bradley, R. (2005). Empirically supported complexity: Rethinking evidence-based practice in psychotherapy. *Current Directions in Psychological Science, 14*(5), 266–271.

Whimster, S., & Lash, S. (2014). *Max Weber, rationality and modernity.* New York: Routledge.

Whitaker, R. (2001). *Mad in America: Bad science, bad medicine, and the enduring mistreatment of the mentally ill.* New York: Basic Books.

Whitley, R. (2014). Beyond critique: Rethinking roles for the anthropology of mental health. *Culture, Medicine, and Psychiatry, 38*, 499–511.

Widiger, T. A. (Ed.). (2015). *The Oxford handbook of the five factor model.* New York: Oxford University Press.

Widiger, T. A., & Oltmanns, J. R. (2017): Neuroticism is a fundamental domain of personality with enormous public health implications. *World Psychiatry, 16*(2), 144–145.

Wiegand, H. F., Hölzel, L., Tüscher, O., Lieb, K., Falkai, P., & Adorjan, K. (2025). Mental health services in Germany–Structures, outcomes and future challenges. *International Review of Psychiatry, 37*(3–4), 253–270.

Wolf, A., Ueda, K., & Hirano, Y. (2021). Recent updates of eye movement abnormalities in patients with schizophrenia: A scoping review. *Psychiatry and Clinical Neurosciences, 75*(3), 82–100.

World Health Organization. (2018). *International classification of diseases,*11th edition. Geneva: World Health Organization.

World Health Organization. (2022). *World mental health report: Transforming mental health for all.* Geneva: World Health Organization.

Yaden, D. B., Goldy, S. P., Weiss, B., & Griffiths, R. R. (2024). Clinically relevant acute subjective effects of psychedelics beyond mystical experience. *Nature Reviews Psychology, 3*(9), 606–621.

Yeo, C., Rennick-Egglestone, S., Armstrong, V., Borg, M., Franklin, D., Klevan, T., . . . & Slade, M. (2022). Uses and misuses of recorded mental health lived experience narratives in healthcare and community settings: Systematic review. *Schizophrenia Bulletin, 48*(1), 134–144.

Young, Z., Moghaddam, N., & Tickle, A. (2020). The efficacy of Cognitive Behavioral Therapy for adults with ADHD: A systematic review and meta-analysis of randomized controlled trials. *Journal of Attention Disorders, 24*(6), 875–888.

Zahl, D. L., & Hawton, K. (2004). Repetition of deliberate self-harm and subsequent suicide risk: Long-term follow-up study of 11583 patients. *The British Journal of Psychiatry, 185*(1), 70–75.

Zahn-Waxler, C., Crick, N. R., Shirtcliff, E. A., & Woods, K. E. (2015). The origins and development of psychopathology in females and males. *Developmental psychopathology: Volume one: Theory and method* (pp. 76–138). New York: John Wiley.

Zanarini, M. C. (2018). *In the fullness of time: Recovery from borderline personality disorder.* New York: Oxford University Press.

Zanarini, M. C., Frankenburg, F. R., Dubo, E. D., Sickel, A. E., Trikha, A., Levin, A., & Reynolds, V. (1998). Axis II comorbidity of borderline personality disorder. *Comprehensive Psychiatry, 39*(5), 296–302.

Zhang, L., Li, L., Andell, P., Garcia-Argibay, M., Quinn, P. D., D'Onofrio, B. M., ... & Chang, Z. (2024). Attention-deficit/hyperactivity disorder medications and long-term risk of cardiovascular diseases. *JAMA Psychiatry, 81*(2), 178–187.

Zimmerman, M. (2021). Why hierarchical dimensional approaches to classification will fail to transform diagnosis in psychiatry. *World Psychiatry, 20*(1), 70.

Zimmerman, M., Rothschild, L., & Chelminski, I. (2005). The prevalence of DSM-IV personality disorders in psychiatric outpatients. *American Journal of Psychiatry, 162*(10), 1911–1918.

Index

For EU product safety concerns, contact us at Calle de José Abascal, 56–1°, 28003 Madrid, Spain or eugpsr@cambridge.org.

www.ingramcontent.com/pod-product-compliance
Ingram Content Group UK Ltd.
Pitfield, Milton Keynes, MK11 3LW, UK
UKHW020106040726

472853UK00009B/385